Lectin-Free Cookbook

The Official Lectin-Free Diet Recipes

<u>Martin Harris</u>

MARTIN HARRIS

LECTIN FREE

COOKBOOK

THE OFFICIAL LECTIN-FREE DIET RECIPES

Table of Contents

original author of this work can be in any fashion deemed liable for any hardship or damages that may befall them after undertaking information described herein.

Additionally, the information in the following pages is intended only for informational purposes and should thus be thought of as universal. As befitting its nature, it is presented without assurance regarding its prolonged validity or interim quality. Trademarks that are mentioned are done without written consent and can in no way be considered an endorsement from the trademark holder.

INTRODUCTION

There are so many different diet regimens that promise to make people lose weight or have better health. But don't you know that even if you are eating healthily, your body is still prone to inflammation, especially if you eat the wrong food? This is where the Lectin-Free Diet comes in. Recently, there has been a growing campaign for this diet to spare consumers the health challenges that are associated with consuming some types of food that are rich in lectin. There is a long list of foods with low lectin content and are, therefore, safe for consumption. This book is designed to help you consume lectin-free foods without going through the conventional rigor of food preparation. With the simple rules, advice, and delicious recipes given in this book, you can prepare a wide range of lectin-free meals without subjecting yourself to too much stress. Many scientists agree that lectins are harmful and can cause different immune system responses. Older studies in the literature claim that consumption of lectin can cause autoimmune diseases such as diabetes, celiac disease, and rheumatoid arthritis. It is also linked to other conditions such as heart disease, cancer, and depression. By following a lectin-free diet, you can lower the risk of severe inflammatory responses in the body. Below are the benefits of a lectin-free diet.

Eating foods that contain lectins can cause gastric distress among very many people. As lectin is not digestible, it binds to the cell membranes of the lining of the digestive tract. Once it latches onto the cell membrane, it disrupts metabolism and causes further damage to the stomach. By restricting the consumption of lectin, it will not only benefit people with food sensitivities but people in general. Although cooking can destroy most lectin in food, it is important to avoid eating raw or undercooked beans, especially kidney beans, because they are very toxic due to their high levels of lectin. By following a lectin-free diet, you don't expose your body to potentially toxic foods. Several studies on laboratory animals show that consumption of lectin can spike the growth of opportunistic, harmful bacteria in the small intestines and can strip it [intestines] of its mucous defense layer, thus increasing the risk for peptic ulcers. A diet containing lectin can disrupt the physiological functions of the digestive system, especially if lectin is eaten over a long period of time. A lectin-free diet may not be able to restore damage already done, but it can help avoid further damage to your digestive tract.

BREAKFAST RECIPES

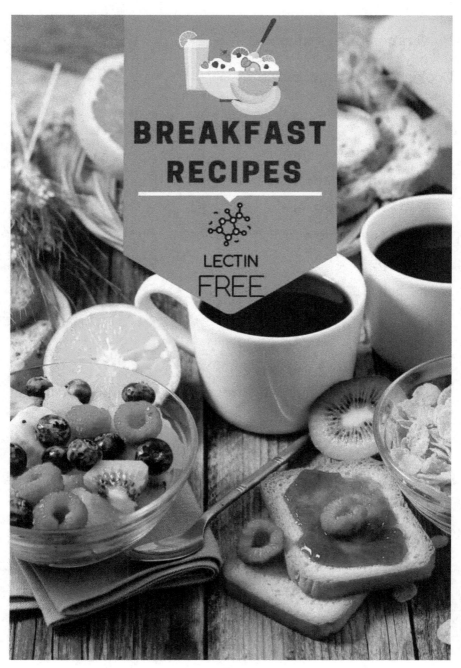

1. <u>Brussels sprouts with Pine Nut</u>

Servings: 4

Preparation time: 5 minutes

Cooking time: 3 minutes

INGREDIENTS

- 1 lb Brussels sprouts
- 1 cup of water
- 1/2 tbsp olive oil
- 1/4 cup pine nuts
- Pepper
- Salt

DIRECTIONS

1. Pour water into the instant pot.
2. Add Brussels sprouts in steamer basket and place basket in the pot.
3. Seal pot with lid and cook on manual high pressure for 3 minutes.
4. Release pressure using the quick release method. Open the lid carefully.
5. Season with pepper and salt. Drizzle with olive oil.
6. Sprinkle pine nuts and serve.

NUTRITION VALUES: Calories: 121; Total Fat: 8g; Saturated Fat: 0.8g; Protein: 5g; Carbs: 11.4g; Fiber: 4.6g; Sugar: 2.8g

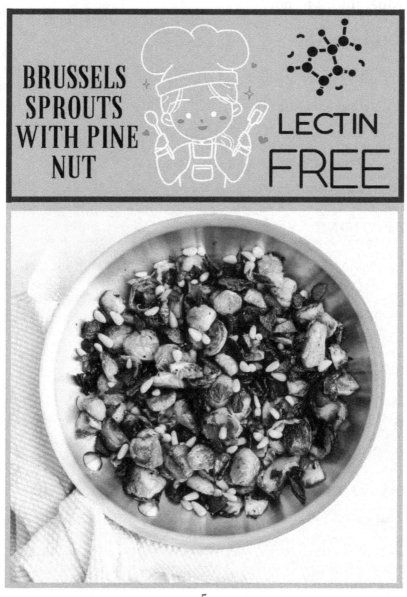

2. <u>Healthy Carrot with Raisins</u>

Servings: 4

Preparation time: 5 minutes

Cooking time: 3 minutes

INGREDIENTS

- 1 lb carrots, peeled and sliced
- 1 tbsp coconut oil
- 1 cup of water
- 3 tbsp raisins
- 1/2 tsp pepper

DIRECTIONS

1. Add water, carrots, and raisins into the instant pot.
2. Seal pot with lid and cook on high for 3 minutes.
3. Release pressure using the quick release method than open lid carefully.
4. Drain carrot well and transfer in a bowl.
5. Add coconut oil in a bowl and toss well until oil is melted.
6. Season with black pepper.
7. Serve and enjoy.

NUTRITION VALUES: Calories: 97; Total Fat: 3.4g; Saturated Fat: 2.9g; Protein: 1.2g; Carbs: 16.7g; Fiber: 3.1g; Sugar: 9.6g

HEALTHY CARROT WITH RAISINS

LECTIN FREE

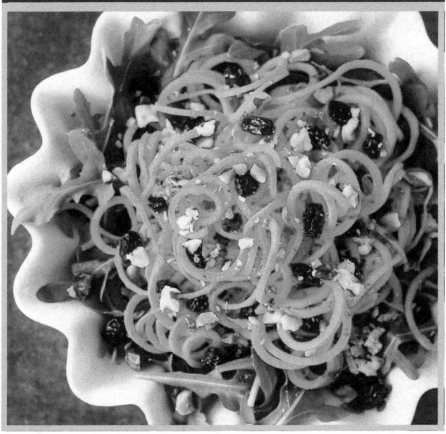

3. <u>**Delicious Korean Egg**</u>

Servings: 1

Preparation time: 5 minutes

Cooking time: 5 minutes

INGREDIENTS

- 1 egg
- 1/8 tsp sesame seeds
- 1 tsp scallions, chopped
- 1/3 cup water
- 1/8 tsp garlic powder
- Pepper
- Salt

DIRECTIONS

1. In a small bowl, whisk together egg and water.
2. Strain egg mixture over a fine strainer into a heat safe bowl.
3. Add remaining ingredients and mix well. Set aside.
4. Pour 1 cup water into the instant pot and then place trivet into the pot.
5. Place egg bowl on a trivet. Seal pot with lid and cook on high pressure for 5 minutes.
6. Release pressure using the quick release method than open the lid carefully.
7. Serve and enjoy.

NUTRITION VALUES: Calories: 67; Total Fat: 4.6g; Saturated Fat: 1.4g; Protein: 5.7g; Carbs: 0.9g; Fiber: 0.2g; Sugar: 0.5g

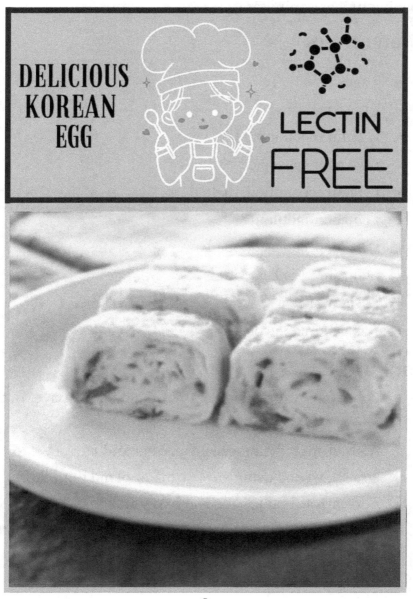

4. **Healthy Carrot Muffins**

Servings: 8

Preparation time: 10 minutes

Cooking time: 20 minutes

INGREDIENTS

- 3 eggs
- 1 1/2 cups water
- 1/2 cup coconut cream
- 1 tsp apple pie spice
- 1/4 cup coconut oil, melted
- 1 cup almond flour
- 1/2 cup pecans, chopped
- 1 cup shredded carrot
- 1/3 cup Truvia
- 1 tsp baking powder

DIRECTIONS

1. Pour water into the instant pot then place a trivet in the pot.
2. Add all ingredients except pecans and carrots into the large bowl and using electric mixer blend until fluffy.
3. Add carrots and pecans and fold well.
4. Pour batter into the silicone muffin cups and place on top of the trivet.
5. Seal pot with lid and cook on high for 20 minutes.

6. Release pressure using quick release method than open the lid.

7. Serve and enjoy.

NUTRITION VALUES: Calories: 256; Total Fat: 24.6g; Saturated Fat: 10.6g; Protein: 6.3g; Carbs: 9.9g; Fiber: 3g; Sugar: 5.2g

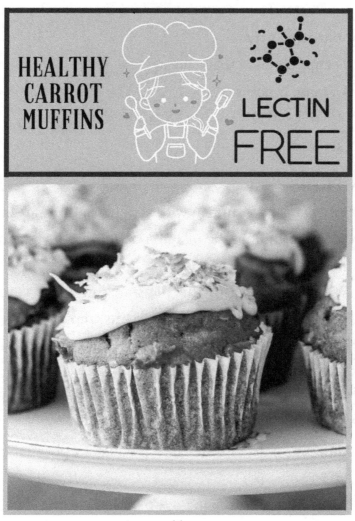

5. <u>Hearty Mushroom Frittata</u>

Servings: 4

Preparation time: 10 minutes

Cooking time: 30 minutes

INGREDIENTS

- 4 pastured large eggs
- 1 tsp dried thyme
- ½ cup coconut cream
- 8 oz mushrooms, sliced
- 1 tbsp olive oil
- 1 tsp salt

DIRECTIONS

1. Spray spring-form pan with cooking spray and set aside.
2. Add olive oil into the instant pot and set the pot on sauté mode.
3. Add mushrooms to the pot and sauté for 5 minutes. Transfer sautéed mushroom to the prepared pan.
4. In a large bowl, whisk eggs and coconut cream until light. Add thyme and salt and mix well.
5. Pour egg mixture into the pan over sautéed mushrooms. Cover pan with foil.
6. Pour 1 ½ cups of water into the instant pot then place a trivet in the pot.
7. Place spring-form pan on top of the trivet.

8. Seal pot with lid and cook on manual high pressure for 25 minutes.
9. Allow to release pressure naturally for 10 minutes then release using the quick release method.
10. Carefully remove the pan from the pot.
11. Slice and serve.

NUTRITION VALUES: Calories: 183; Total Fat: 15.8g; Saturated Fat: 8.4g; Protein: 8.8g; Carbs: 4.1g; Fiber: 1.3g; Sugar: 2.4g

Hearty Mushroom Frittata

LECTIN FREE

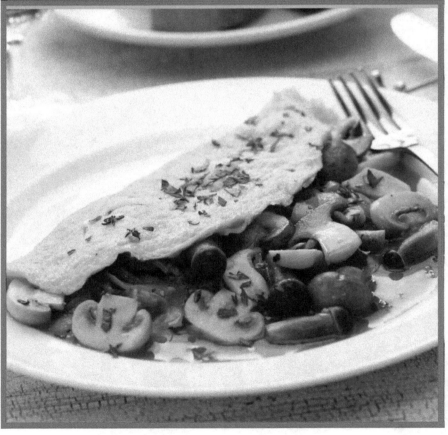

6. <u>Scrambled Eggs</u>

Servings: 4

Preparation time: 10 minutes

Cooking time: 6 minutes

INGREDIENTS

- 4 pastured eggs
- ½ tsp allspice
- 2 tsp cinnamon
- 2 tbsp olive oil
- ¼ tsp black pepper
- 1/8 tsp salt

DIRECTIONS

1. Add olive oil into the instant pot and set the pot on sauté mode.
2. In a mixing bowl, add eggs and beat until light.
3. Add allspice, cinnamon, pepper, and salt.
4. Add egg mixture to the pot and cook for 2 minutes. Scramble the eggs using a spatula.
5. Seal pot with lid and cook on manual high pressure for 4 minutes.
6. Release pressure using the quick release method than open the lid.
7. Serve and enjoy.

NUTRITION VALUES: Calories: 134; Total Fat: 11.5g; Saturated Fat: 2.5g; Protein: 6.1g; Carbs: 2.2g; Fiber: 0.7g; Sugar: 0g

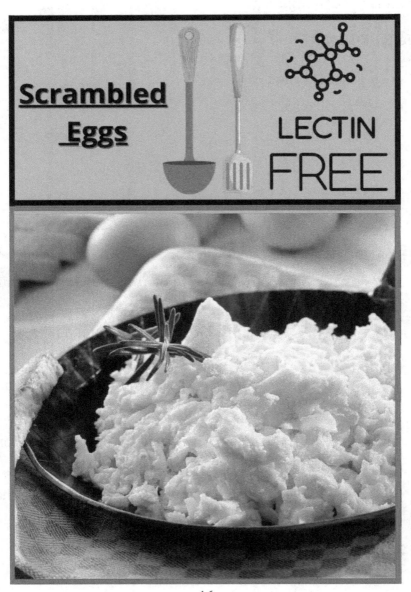

7. __Broccoli Frittata__

Servings: 4

Preparation time: 10 minutes

Cooking time: 20 minutes

INGREDIENTS
- 6 pastured eggs
- 1/3 cup coconut milk
- ½ cup broccoli florets, chopped
- ¼ cup fresh dill, chopped
- 1/3 cup goat cheese, crumbled
- Pepper
- Salt

DIRECTIONS
1. In a bowl, beat eggs, with broccoli, coconut milk, dill, and goat cheese.
2. Transfer egg mixture into a greased 7-inch spring-form pan. Cover pan with foil.
3. Pour 2 cups of water into the instant pot then place a trivet in the pot.
4. Place spring-form pan on top of the trivet.
5. Seal pot with lid and cook on manual high pressure for 20 minutes.

6. Allow to release pressure naturally for 10 minutes then release using the quick release method.

7. Serve and enjoy. **NUTRITION VALUES:** Calories: 223; Total Fat: 16.3g; Saturated Fat: 9.5g; Protein: 14.4g; Carbs: 5.8g; Fiber: 1.2g; Sugar: 0.9g

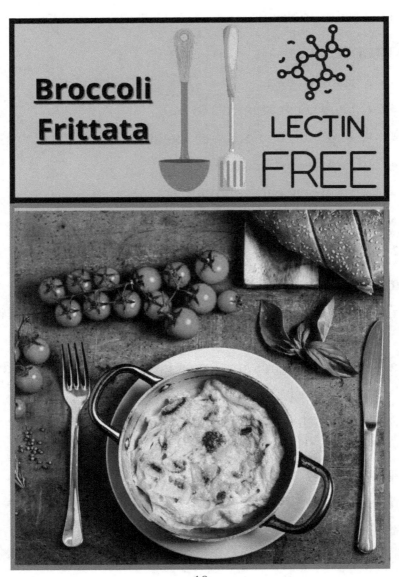

8. <u>**Spinach Frittata**</u>

Servings: 6

Preparation time: 10 minutes

Cooking time: 10 minutes

INGREDIENTS

- 7 pastured large eggs
- 1 cup of water
- 1 ½ cups baby spinach, chopped
- ½ tsp nutmeg, grated
- 2 tbsp coconut cream
- Pepper
- Salt

DIRECTIONS

1. In a bowl, beat eggs with nutmeg, coconut cream, pepper, and salt until smooth.
2. Add spinach and stir well.
3. Spray 7-inch spring-form pan with cooking spray.
4. Pour egg mixture into the prepared pan.
5. Pour 1 cup of water into the instant pot then place a trivet in the pot.
6. Place pan on top of the trivet.
7. Seal pot with lid and cook on high pressure for 10 minutes.

8. Release pressure using the quick release method than open the lid.

9. Serve and enjoy.

NUTRITION VALUES: Calories: 96; Total Fat: 6.5g; Saturated Fat: 2.8g; Protein:7.4g; Carbs: 1.8g; Fiber: 0.3g; Sugar: 0.3g

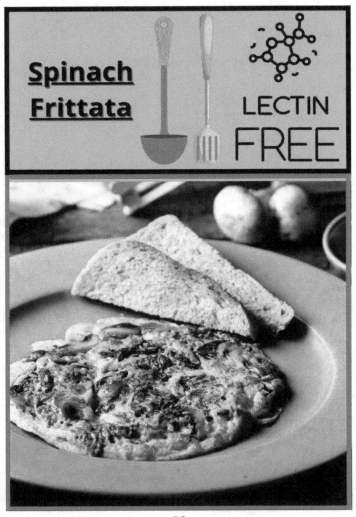

9. Spinach Mushroom Frittata

Servings: 6

Preparation time: 10 minutes

Cooking time: 30 minutes

INGREDIENTS

- 8 pastured eggs
- 2 tbsp coconut milk
- 1 tbsp fresh lemon juice
- ¼ cup goat cheese, crumbled
- 6 oz baby spinach, rinsed
- 2 garlic cloves, minced
- ½ onion, chopped
- 8 oz mushrooms, sliced
- 2 tbsp olive oil
- ¼ tsp black pepper
- Salt

DIRECTIONS

1. Heat olive oil in a pan over medium-high heat.
2. Add onion and mushrooms to the pan and sauté for 3 minutes.
3. Add garlic, lemon juice, pepper, and salt and sauté for 30 seconds.
4. In a large bowl, beat eggs.

5. Add cheese, milk, and mushrooms mixture to the eggs and stir well.
6. Add spinach to the egg mixture and stir well.
7. Pour egg mixture into the 7-inch greased pan.
8. Pour 2 cups of water into the instant pot then place a trivet in the pot.
9. Place pan on top of the trivet.
10. Seal pot with lid and cook on manual high pressure for 25 minutes.
11. Allow to release pressure naturally for 10 minutes then release using the quick release method.
12. Serve and enjoy.

NUTRITION VALUES: Calories: 285; Total Fat: 21.4g; Saturated Fat: 9.7g; Protein: 18.3g; Carbs: 6.5g; Fiber: 1.4g; Sugar: 1.4g

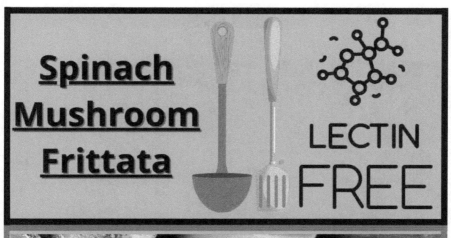

Spinach Mushroom Frittata

LECTIN FREE

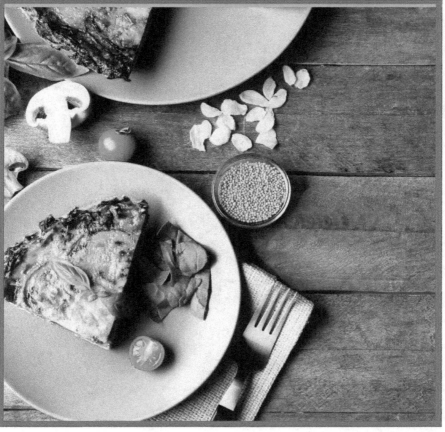

MAINS

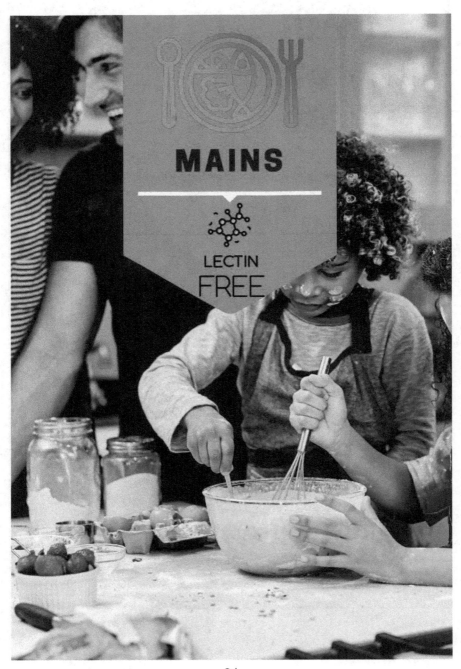

10. **Mexican Garlic and Kale Medley:**

Servings: 3

Cooking time: 5 hours

NUTRITION VALUES: Calories: 52 Protein: 3grams Fat: 1gramsCarbohydrates: 11grams

INGREDIENTS

- 4 bunch kale, washed, stemmed and cut into large pieces
- 2 onions, chopped
- 8 garlic cloves, minced
- 2 jalapeno peppers, minced
- 4 large red bell peppers, deseeded, sliced
- 1 tablespoon chili powder
- ½ teaspoon salt
- 1/8 teaspoon freshly ground black pepper

DIRECTIONS

1. Add kale, onions, jalapeno peppers, garlic, bell pepper to your slow cooker
2. Sprinkle chili powder, salt, and pepper, and stir
3. Cover with lid and cook on LOW for 4-5 hours until the kale is tender
4. Serve and enjoy!

11. <u>**Syrian-Style Shakriyeh lamb Yogurt Stew:**</u>

Servings: 4

Cooking time: 1 hour

NUTRITION VALUES: Calories: 459 Protein: 53grams Fat: 17gramsCarbohydrates: 17grams

INGREDIENTS

- 2 pounds boneless lamb shoulder, cut into bite-sized pieces
- 8 cups homemade low-sodium chicken broth or water
- 1 large red onion or yellow onion, finely chopped
- 4 tablespoons of sea salt, divided
- 2 tablespoons arrowroot powder
- 4 tablespoons toasted pine units (for garnishing
- 2 cups unsweetened coconut yogurt or goat yogurt

DIRECTIONS

1. Add lamb pieces, chicken broth, and 2 tablespoons of the salt to the instant pot
2. Lock, seal the lid. Press the "Manual" button. Cook on HIGH 40 minutes
3. When done, quick release or naturally release pressure remove the lid.
4. Remove lamb pieces from instant pot
5. In a blender, combine yogurt, salt, arrowroot powder. Pulse until smooth.

6. Press "State" function. Slowly stir in yogurt mixture with liquid. Simmer until it combines and thickens. Return cooked lamed to pot. Simmer 3 minutes.

7. Transfer lamb and sauce to a serving platter. Garnish with toasted pine nuts.serve.

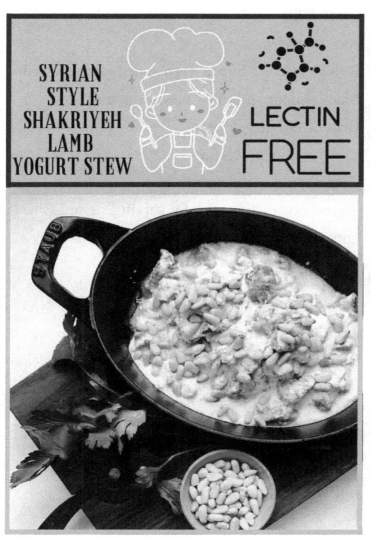

SYRIAN STYLE SHAKRIYEH LAMB YOGURT STEW · LECTIN FREE

12. Creamy Swiss chard Patties with Goat Cheese:

Servings: 4

Cooking time: 32minutes

NUTRITION VALUES: Calories: 66.9 Protein: 3.0grams Fat: 3.5gramsCarbohydrates: 7.7grams

INGREDIENTS

- Garlic – 3cloves, chopped
- Swiss chard – a bunch, torn and stems removed
- Black pepper and salt – according to taste
- Ground cumin – ½ tsp.
- Cassava flour – ½ cup
- Goat cheese – 2 ounces
- Source cream – enough for serving, organic
- Olive oil – 4 tbsp., extra virgin

DIRECTIONS

1. In a blender, prepare a pulse of garlic, Swiss chard, cumin, pepper as well as salt. Collect in a bowl.
2. Include goat cheese in this mixture of Swiss chard. Use another bowl to mix everything properly.
3. Prepare medium-sized patties with this mixture. Keep your patties not thicker than ¼ inch.
4. Use a nonstick pan to cook the patties using heated olive oil.

5. Keep the heat medium-high and cook each side of the patties for about 2 to 4 minutes until you get a brown color.
6. Serve with sour cream.

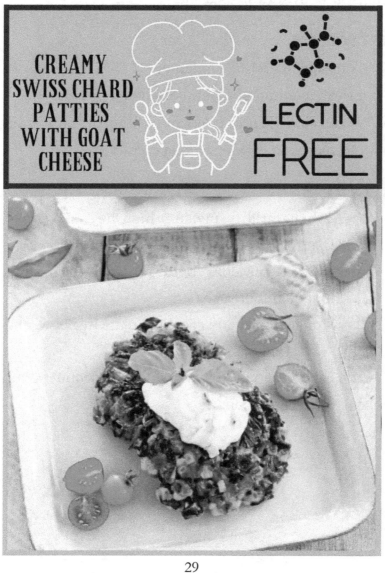

CREAMY SWISS CHARD PATTIES WITH GOAT CHEESE

LECTIN FREE

13. Grilled Peaches:

Servings: 8

Cooking time: 14minutes

NUTRITION VALUES: Calories: 69 Protein: 0.9grams Fat: 5.1gramsCarbohydrates: 5.3grams

INGREDIENTS

- ¼ teaspoon ground cinnamon
- 2 fresh medium peaches, halved and pitted
- ¼ cup chilled coconut cream, whipped
- 1 ½ teaspoon organic vanilla extract

DIRECTIONS

1. Preheat the grill to medium-high heat and grease the grill grate
2. Arrange the peaches onto prepared grill and grill for about 7 minutes per side
3. Put vanilla extract and coconut cream in a bowl and beat until well combined.
4. Top each peach piece with whipped coconut cream and dust with cinnamon.

GRILLED PEACHES

LECTIN FREE

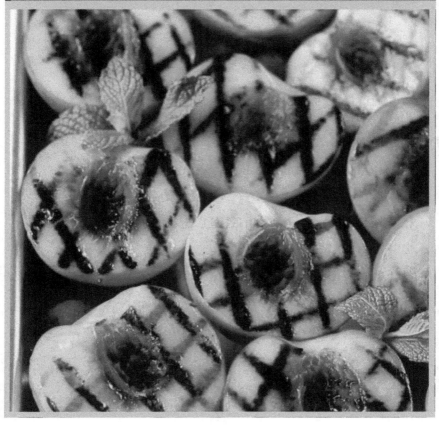

14. Authentic Charred Soup:

Servings: 4

Cooking time: 3 hours 5minutes

NUTRITION VALUES: Calories: 284 Protein: 15grams Fat: 19gramsCarbohydrates: 13grams

INGREDIENTS

- 2 and ½ cup Swiss chard, chopped
- 2 tablespoons ginger, minced
- 1 cup onion, chopped
- 1 teaspoon oregano
- Salt as needed
- Red chili flakes as needed

DIRECTIONS

1. Add the listed ingredients your slow cooker
2. Add enough water to cover the ingredients
3. Close lid and cook on MEDIUM for 3 hours
4. Let it sit for a while
5. Open aid and use an immersion blender to blend the soup into a creamy texture
6. Stir and enjoy with more seasoning if needed.

15. Balsamic Brussels sprouts:

Servings: 4

Cooking time: 23minutes

NUTRITION VALUES: Calories: 206 Protein: 14.5grams Fat: 12.3gramsCarbohydrates: 10.9grams

INGREDIENTS

- 2 cups water
- 1 pound fresh organic Brussels sprouts, trimmed, halved
- 6 slices of bacon, chopped
- 4 tablespoons fresh chives, finely chopped
- 2 tablespoons balsamic vinegar
- Pinch of salt, pepper

DIRECTIONS

1. Add water and steamer basket to instant pot
2. Place Brussels sprouts on top of the steamer basket
3. Close, seal the lid. Press the "manual" button. Cook on HIGH 2 minutes
4. When done, quick release pressure. Remove the lid.
5. Transfer Brussels sprouts to a bowl. remove steamer basket discard the water
6. Press "Sauté" function. Add chopped bacon. Cook until brown.

7. While pot is still hot, return Brussels sprouts to the pot with bacon. Stir in balsamic vinegar, salt, pepper. Transfer to platter. Garnish with fresh chives. Serve.

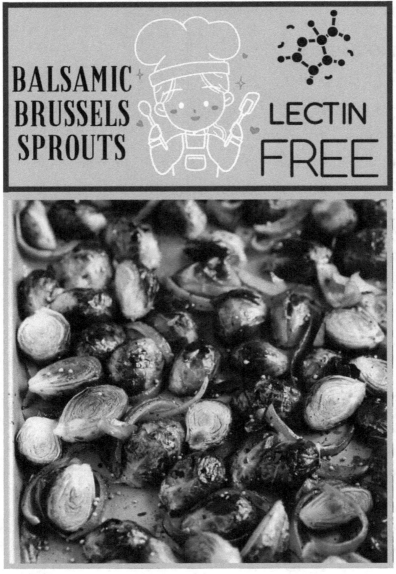

16. Tangy Mushroom Grilled Chicken with Shredded Cauliflower:

Servings: 4

Cooking time: 46minutes

NUTRITION VALUES: Calories: 118.2 Protein: 4.4grams Fat: 4.3gramsCarbohydrates: 17.3grams

INGREDIENTS

- Lime zest – 1 lime
- Cauliflower – 1 head, shredded
- Pasture – fed chicken things – ¾ pound, skin, and bones removed, small pieces
- Red onion – 1, small
- Portabella mushroom – 2, small pieces
- Olive oil – 2 tbsp., extra virgin
- Limes – 2, cut to make 8 pieces
- Sea salt
- Ground cumin – ½ tsp.
- Oil for grilling
- Black pepper – according to taste
- Lime wedges – for serving

DIRECTIONS

1. Prepare your grill by preheating, then, place the grill pan, keeping the heat to medium.

2. Put the shredded cauliflower in a dish and cover. Shift this dish to your microwave and cook for about 4 to 5 minutes. Set aside for 3 minutes, then, use a check until it becomes fluffy.

3. Include the lime zest in the fluffed cauliflower and mix properly.

4. Now, take a large bowl to mix together the mushroom, chicken, limes, onion, cumin, oil, pepper and salt

5. Put oil in the heated pan and shift vegetables and chicken mixture on the grilling pan. Cook by stirring from time to time. This will take about 16 to 18 minutes to cook the chicken pieces and make the onion pieces tender.

6. Use lime wedges and prepare plates with cauliflower and cooked mushroom and chicken.

17. Orange Shredded Pork:

Servings: 8

Cooking time: 1 hour 30minutes

NUTRITION VALUES: Calories: 295 Protein: 45.9grams Fat: 6.1gramsCarbohydrates: 9.5grams

INGREDIENTS

- 3 pounds boneless pork butt, cut into 3 equal sized pieces
- 1 ½ cups fresh orange juice
- 1 medium sweet onion, finely chopped
- 4 dried anchor chilies, stemmed, seeded
- 4 garlic cloves, minced
- 2/3 cups organic apple cider vinegar
- ½ cup fresh parsley, finely chopped
- 1 teaspoon dried oregano
- ½ teaspoon organic ground cumin
- Pinch of sea salt, pepper

DIRECTIONS

1. Add the orange juice and pork pieces to your instant pot
2. Lock, seal the lid .press"manual"button.cook on HIGH 50 minutes at
3. When done naturally release pressure. remove the lid
4. Transfer pork pieces to a serving platter. Shred using two forks. Set aside.

5. In a blender, combine onion, ancho chilies, garlic cloves apple cider vinegar, parsley, oregano, ground cumin, salt, and black pepper. Blend until smooth.

6. Press "state" function on instant pot. Set to low. Pour in the sauce. Simmer a couple of minutes until thickens, stressing occasionally.

7. Stir in shredded pork to coat evenly. Transfer to platter service.

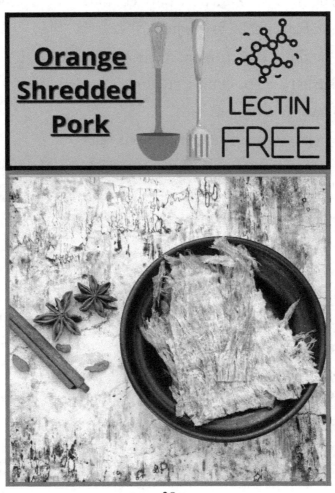

18. Shirataki Rice and Pastured Chicken Soup:

Servings: 4

Cooking time: 21minutes

NUTRITION VALUES: Calories: 204.7 Protein: 25.0grams
Fat: 5.2gramsCarbohydrates: 13.4grams

INGREDIENTS

- Onion – 1 large, sliced
- Shirataki rice – 1 pack
- Garlic -4 cloves, chopped
- Olive oil -3 tbsp.
- Broth -6 cups
- Rosemary- 1 sprig
- Pastured chicken -12 ounces, cooked, shredded
- Black pepper and salt –according to taste
- Parmigiano-Reggiano –to serve, grated, lection free
- Baby spinach - 5 ounces

DIRECTIONS

1. Use warm water to rinse and drain shirataki rice
2. Heat your large pot over medium heat. Include oil and let it get wormed. Then, put onion and brown for about 7 to 8 minutes. Add rosemary and garlic and let the mixture cook for 2 minutes more

3. After getting the garlic fragrance, include salt according to taste along with pepper oil the mixture then simmer for about 12 to 15 minutes.

4. Mix spinach, rice, and shredded chicken and stir properly. Stir cook for about 4 to 5 minutes and serve with parmigiana on the top

5. Serve!

19. Hearty broccoli:

Servings: 6

Cooking time: 15minutes

NUTRITION VALUES: Calories: 116 Protein: 4.1grams Fat: 7.1gramsCarbohydrates: 12.1grams

INGREDIENTS

- 1 ½ tablespoon coconut oil
- 1 ½ pound fresh broccoli florets
- 1 ½ tablespoons fresh ginger, minced
- 1 ½ teaspoon cumin seeds
- ¾ cup unsweetened coconut flakes
- 3 teaspoon curry powder
- 3 tablespoon filtered water
- ¾ small yellow onion sliced thinly

DIRECTIONS

1. Heat a large non-stick skillet over medium heat and add coconut flakes
2. Cook for about 4 minutes and dish out in a bowl
3. Heat oil in the same skillet and add of the ingredients except for broccoli
4. Sauté for about 2 minutes and add water and broccoli
5. Stir to combine and enhance the heat to medium-high
6. Cover and cook for about 4 minutes
7. Top with toasted coconut flakes and serve

Hearty Broccoli

LECTIN FREE

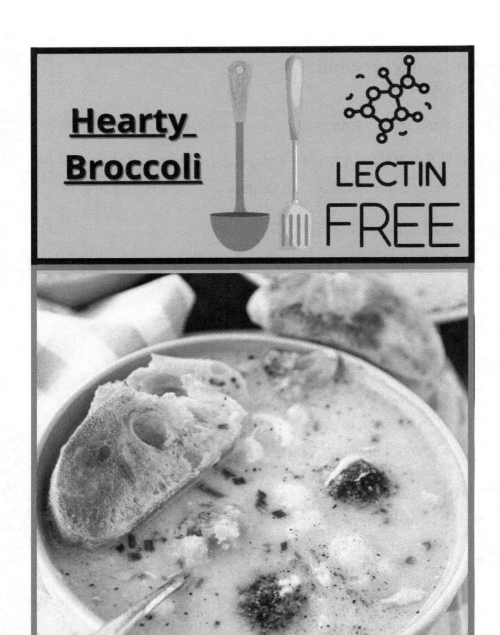

20. **Beet and Onion Delight:**

Servings: 6

Cooking time: 5-7 hours

NUTRITION VALUES: Calories: 140 Protein: 2grams Fat: 4gramsCarbohydrates: 27gram

INGREDIENTS

- 10 medium beets, peeled and diced
- 3 red onions, chopped
- 4 garlic cloves, minced
- 2 tablespoons stevia
- 1/3 cup lemon juice
- 1 cup water
- 2 tablespoons melted coconut oil
- 3 tablespoons arrowroot
- ½ teaspoon salt

DIRECTIONS

1. Add beets, onions, and garlic to your Slow cooker
2. Take a medium bowl and add stevia, lemon juice, coconut oil, water, arrowroot, salt and stir until combined
3. Pour mixture over beets
4. Cover and cook for 5-7 hours until the beets are tender
5. Enjoy!

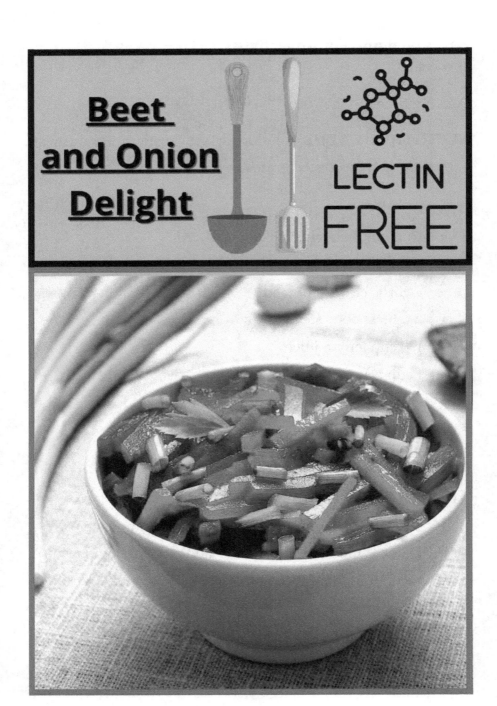

Beet and Onion Delight

LECTIN FREE

21. <u>Wine and Coffee Beef Stew:</u>

Servings: 8

Cooking time: 30minutes

NUTRITION VALUES: Calories: 242 Protein: 30.1grams Fat: 13.28gramsCarbohydrates: 1.35grams

INGREDIENTS

- 2 ½ pounds organic grass-fed beef chuck stew meat, cut into bite-sized chunks
- 3 tablespoons olive oil, coconut oil avocado oil, or ghee
- 2 tablespoons organic capers,2 garlic cloves, minced
- 3 cups of homemade freshly brewed coffee
- 1 cup of homemade organic low-sodium beef bone broth
- 2 cups of fresh organic mushroom, sliced
- 2/3 cups organic red cooking wine
- 1 medium onion, finely chopped
- 2 tablespoons arrowroot powder
- Pinch of salt pepper

DIRECTIONS

1. Press "sauté" function on instant pot. Add the oil
2. Once hot, working in batches if necessary, add stewing beef, sear on all sides. Remove and set aside.

3. Add garlic, onion, and mushroom to instant pot. Cook until slightly softened, stirring occasionally. Turn off "Sauté" function on your instant pot.

4. Return browned stew meat. Stir in capers, brewed coffee, beef broth, red cooking wine, salt, and pepper.

5. Lock, seal the lid. Press the "Manual" button. Cook on high 25 minutes.

6. When done, allow full natural release. Remove the lid.

7. Press "Sauté" function on instant pot. Sprinkle the arrowroot powder and allow simmering until the liquid is reduced and thickens. Transfer to platter and serve.

22. **Cassava Cinnamon Pancakes:**

Servings: 4

Cooking time: 36minutes

NUTRITION VALUES: Calories: 107 Protein: 1grams Fat: 0gramsCarbohydrates: 12grams

INGREDIENTS

- Fruit sweetener – 2 tbsp.
- Cassava flour – 1 cup
- Cinnamon – 1 tsp., more for topping
- Baking powder -1 tbsp.
- Nutmeg – 1/8 Tsp.
- Sea salt – ¼ tsp.
- Vanilla extract – ½ tsp.
- Kefir of Goats buttermilk – 1 ¼ cup, keep in the room temperature
- Large pasture – fed eggs – 2 pcs
- Water – ¼ cup
- Melted butter – 3 tbsp., more, use lection free butter

DIRECTIONS

1. Prepare your griddle for cooking by preheating. Make sure the griddle is nonstick
2. In a large bowl, mix sweetener, flour, cinnamon, nutmeg, baking powder, and sea salt.

3. Then, mix kefir, eggs, water, and vanilla in a different bowl. Also, include butter and whisk in this mixture

4. Take a new large bowl to mix the wet and the dry mixtures. Whisk thoroughly to until it turns into a smooth texture.

5. Use a measuring cup and pour up to ¼ cup of better in the preheated griddle. Cook pancakes until you see bubbles breaking on the surface and the color getting golden brown. Cook for 2 minutes on one side and then cook for extra minutes after pepping.

6. Make all pancakes and serve warm with cinnamon and butter.

23. **Colorful Beet Pesto:**

Servings: 6

Cooking time: 1 hour

NUTRITION VALUES: Calories: 231 Protein: 5.8grams Fat: 16.7gramsCarbohydrates: 18.8gram

INGREDIENTS

For pesto:

- 8 cups fresh basil leaves
- Salt and freshly ground black pepper, to taste
- 3 large garlic cloves, chopped
- ½ cup pine nuts, chopped roughly
- 1/3 cup extra-virgin olive oil

For cooking:

- 3 tablespoons olive oil
- 6 cups fresh kale, chopped
- 6 medium beets, trimmed, peeled and spiraled with blade C

DIRECTIONS

1. Preheat the oven to 430 degrees F and grease a large baking sheet
2. Add all the pesto ingredients in food processor except oil and pulse until smooth
3. Add olive oil and process again and set aside

4. Place beet in a prepared baking sheet and sprinkle with oil, sea salt, and black pepper.

5. Roast for about 10 minutes and dish in a large bowl.

6. Add kale and pesto and toss well.

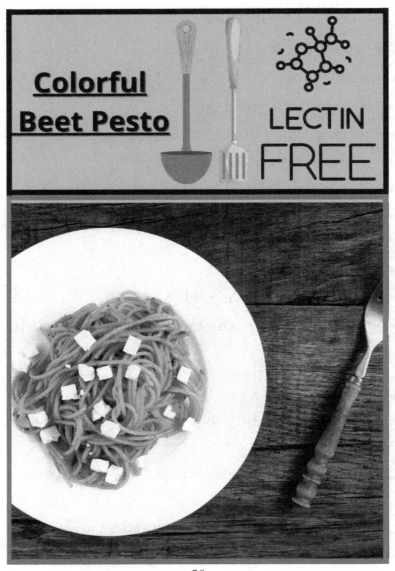

SEAFOOD

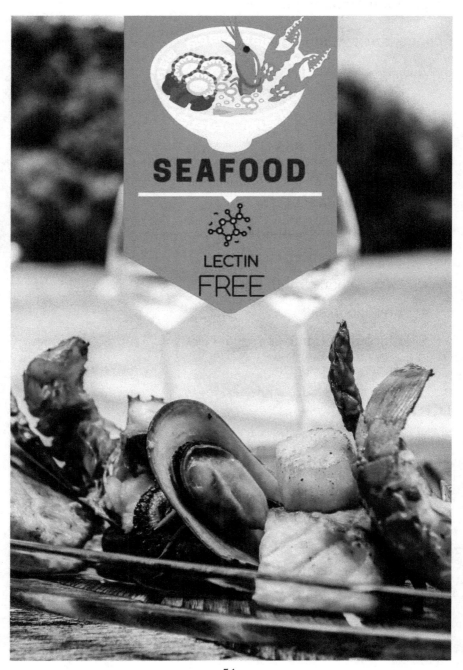

24.   **Fish Casserole**

Preparation Time: 15 minutes

Cooking time: 35 minutes

Servings:4

INGREDIENTS

- 1 cup broccoli florets
- ½ cup heavy cream
- 6 oz Cheddar cheese
- 10 oz cod fillet, chopped
- 1 oz green onion, chopped
- ¾ teaspoon chili flakes
- 1 teaspoon salt
- 1 tablespoon butter
- 1 teaspoon capers

DIRECTIONS

1. Chop the broccoli florets roughly.
2. Shred Cheddar cheese.
3. Sprinkle the chopped cod fillet with the chili flakes and salt. Mix up well.
4. Spread the casserole dish with the butter. Place the chopped cod inside.
5. Then sprinkle the fish with capers and chopped broccoli florets.
6. Arrange the chopped green onion over the broccoli.

7. Then add shredded cheese and heavy cream.

8. Preheat the oven to 375F and place the casserole inside.

9. Cook it for 35 minutes.

NUTRITION VALUES: Calories 319, Fat 23.3, Fiber 0.8, Carbs 3.1, Protein 25.1

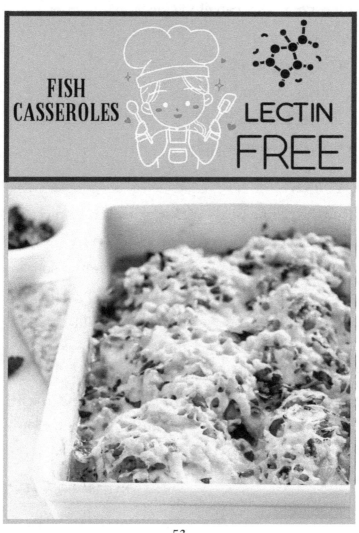

25.   **Mexican Style Tilapia**

Preparation Time: 20 minutes

Cooking time: 7 minutes

Servings:2

INGREDIENTS

- 1 teaspoon Mexican chili spices
- 2 tilapia fillets
- ¾ teaspoon dried rosemary
- 1 tablespoon lime juice
- 1 tablespoon canola oil
- 1 teaspoon sour cream

DIRECTIONS

1. Rub the tilapia fillets with Mexican chili spices and dried rosemary.
2. Then sprinkle the fish with lime juice and sour cream/
3. Massage it well with the help of the fingertips.
4. Brush the fish gently with the canola oil.
5. Let it marinate for 15 minutes.
6. Meanwhile, preheat the grill well.
7. Place the marinated fish in the grill and roast it for 3 minutes from each side or until it is light brown.

NUTRITION VALUES: Calories 161, Fat 8.5, Fiber 0.2, Carbs 0.4, Protein 21.1

MEXICAN STYLE TILAPIA

LECTIN FREE

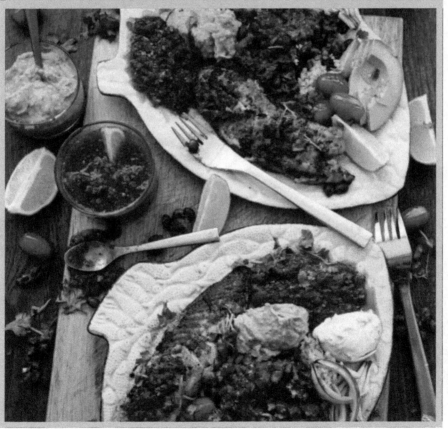

26.   **Rosemary Haddock**

Preparation Time: 15 minutes

Cooking time: 20 minutes

Servings:4

INGREDIENTS

- 1 teaspoon tarragon
- 1 teaspoon dried rosemary
- 1-pound haddock fillet
- ½ teaspoon onion powder
- ¾ teaspoon salt
- 2 tablespoons olive oil
- 1 oz Parmesan, grated
- 1 tablespoon butter

DIRECTIONS

1. Mix up together tarragon, dried rosemary, onion powder, and salt.
2. Sprinkle the haddock fillet with the spice mixture.
3. Then cut it into 4 pieces.
4. Brush the baking dish with the olive oil.
5. Place the haddock fillets inside.
6. Sprinkle the fish with the grated cheese. Add butter.
7. Cook the haddock for 20 minutes in the preheated to the 365F oven.

NUTRITION VALUES: Calories 238, Fat 12.5, Fiber 0.2, Carbs 0.8, Protein 29.9

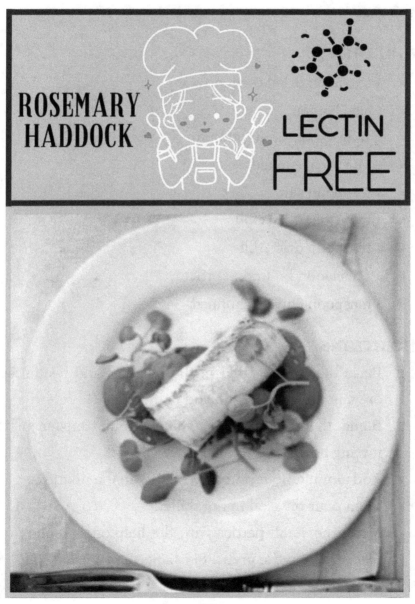

27. Oregano Tuna Patties

Preparation Time: 15 minutes

Cooking time: 5 minutes

Servings:4

INGREDIENTS

- 1 teaspoon dried oregano
- 1 egg, beaten
- 3 tablespoons almond flour
- 10 oz tuna, canned
- 1 teaspoon salt
- 1 tablespoon olive oil
- 1 teaspoon dried dill
- ½ teaspoon ground paprika
- 1 teaspoon chives, chopped

DIRECTIONS

1. Place the canned tuna in the blender, add beaten egg, oregano, salt, dried dill, and paprika,
2. Blend the mixture until smooth and transfer in the mixing bowl.
3. Add almond flour and chives. Mix up the mixture.
4. Then pour olive oil in the skillet.
5. Make the small patties with the help of the spoon and place them in the preheated skillet.

6. Cook the patties for 2 minutes and then flip them onto another side.

7. The cooked tuna patties will have a golden brown color.

NUTRITION VALUES: Calories 300, Fat 20.9, Fiber 2.6, Carbs 5.1, Protein 24.8

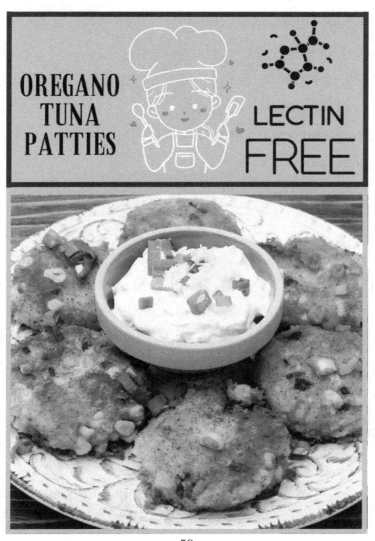

28.   Crab Cakes

Preparation Time: 10 minutes

Cooking time: 6 minutes

Servings:7

INGREDIENTS

- 12 oz crabmeat, chopped
- 1 tablespoon chives, chopped
- ½ teaspoon turmeric
- ½ teaspoon garlic, diced
- 3 tablespoons coconut flour
- 1/3 teaspoon salt
- ½ teaspoon ground black pepper
- 1 tablespoon olive oil
- 1 egg, beaten

DIRECTIONS

1. In the mixing bowl, mix up together chopped crab meat, chives, turmeric, diced garlic, coconut flour, salt, ground black pepper, and beaten egg.
2. Mix up the crab mixture with the help of the spoon.
3. Put olive oil in the pan and bring it to boil.
4. Make the crab cakes with the help of 2 spoons and transfer them in the boiled oil.
5. Cook the crab cakes for 6 minutes (for 3 minutes from each side) over the medium heat.

6. Chill the cooked crab cakes little before serving.

NUTRITION VALUES: Calories 87, Fat 3.3, Fiber 1.4, Carbs 9.3, Protein 5

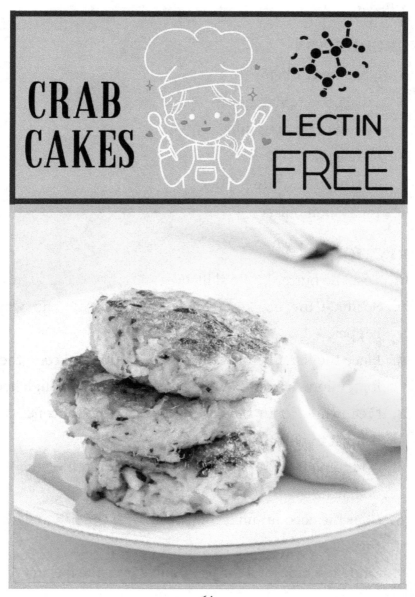

29. Fish Fillets in Tomato Sauce

Preparation Time: 10 minutes

Cooking time: 15 minutes

Servings:4

INGREDIENTS

- 4 mackerel fillets
- 1 teaspoon tomato paste
- ¾ cup of coconut milk
- ½ teaspoon salt
- ¾ teaspoon white pepper
- 1 teaspoon butter

DIRECTIONS

1. Toss the butter in the skillet.
2. Sprinkle the mackerel fillets with the salt and white pepper.
3. Place the fish fillets on the melted butter and cook them for 3 minutes from each side over the medium-high heat.
4. Meanwhile, pour the coconut milk in the saucepan and bring it to boil.
5. Add tomato paste and whisk it until smooth. Bring it to boil again.
6. Pour the coconut mixture (sauce) over the fish and close the lid.
7. Saute the mackerel for 10 minutes over the low heat.

NUTRITION VALUES: Calories 345, Fat 27.4, Fiber 1.1, Carbs 3, Protein 22.1

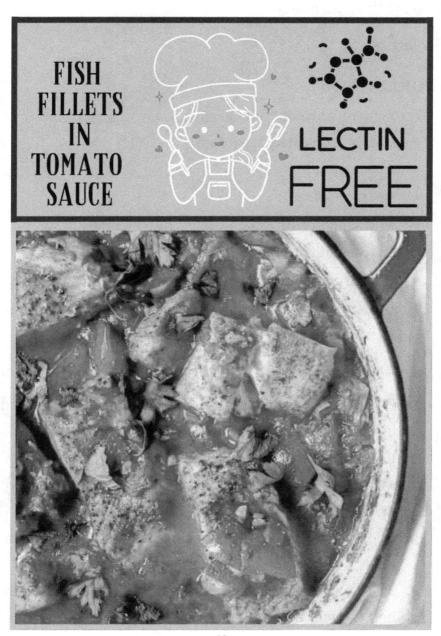

30.   Stuffed Mushroom Caps with Halibut

Preparation Time: 15 minutes

Cooking time: 20 minutes

Servings:5

INGREDIENTS

- 1 cup mushroom caps
- ½ teaspoon dried marjoram
- 10 oz halibut
- ½ onion, diced
- ¾ teaspoon chili flakes
- ½ teaspoon dried oregano
- 1 tablespoon butter
- 1 teaspoon olive oil
- ½ teaspoon garlic powder

DIRECTIONS

1. Finely chop the halibut and mix it up with the diced onion, chili flakes, dried oregano, and garlic powder. Add dried marjoram.
2. Mix up the mixture and transfer it in the pan. Add olive oil.
3. Cook the fish mixture for 10 minutes over the medium heat.
4. Then fill the mushroom caps with the halibut mixture and transfer them in the baking tray.

5. Cover the tray with foil and secure the edges.

6. Cook the mushroom caps for 10 minutes at 370F.

7. When the time is over, let the mushroom caps rest for 10 minutes in the switched off oven.

8. Then discard the foil and transfer the mushrooms in the serving plates.

NUTRITION VALUES: Calories 142, Fat 5.5, Fiber 0.5, Carbs 1.8, Protein 20.7

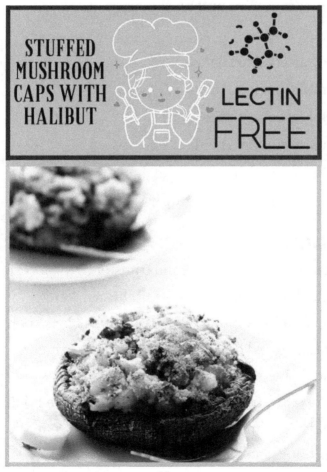

31.<u>Keto Salmon Burger</u>

Preparation Time: 10 minutes

Cooking time: 10 minutes

Servings:4

INGREDIENTS

- 1-pound salmon fillet
- 1 tablespoon almond flour
- ½ teaspoon ground black pepper
- 1 egg, beaten
- ¼ cup coconut flakes
- 1 tablespoon olive oil
- 1 tablespoon chives, chopped
- 1 teaspoon dried dill
- 1 teaspoon dried parsley
- ¼ teaspoon ground ginger

DIRECTIONS

1. Chop the salmon fillet and transfer in the food processor.
2. Blend it for 1 minute or until it is smooth.
3. Then add almond flour, ground black pepper, egg, chives, dried dill, parsley, and ground ginger.
4. Pulse the mixture for 30 seconds.
5. After this, transfer the fish mixture in the mixing bowl.
6. Make the medium size burgers and coat them in the coconut flakes.

7. Preheat the olive oil over the medium heat.

8. Place the salmon burgers in the hot oil and cook them for 4 minutes from each side.

9. The salmon burgers are cooked when they are light brown color.

NUTRITION VALUES: Calories 255, Fat 16.8, Fiber 1.3, Carbs 2.8, Protein 25.2

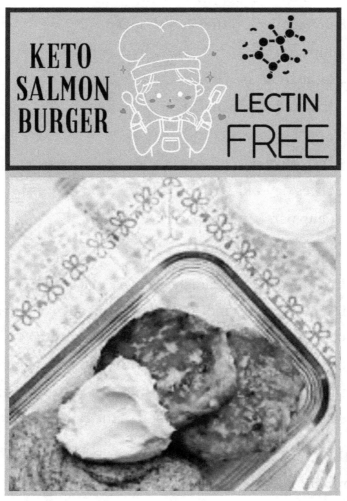

32. __Grilled Salmon with Radish Salad__

Preparation Time: 22 minutes

Servings: 2-4

INGREDIENTS

- 1 lb skinned salmon, cut into 4 steaks each
- 1 cup radishes, sliced
- Salt and black pepper to taste
- 8 green olives, pitted and chopped
- 1 cup arugula
- 2 large tomatoes, diced
- 3 tbsp red wine vinegar
- 2 green onions, sliced
- 3 tbsp olive oil
- 2 slices day-old zero carb bread, cubed
- ¼ cup parsley, chopped

DIRECTIONS

1. In a bowl, mix the radishes, olives, black pepper, arugula, tomatoes, wine vinegar, green onion, olive oil, bread, and parsley. Let sit for the flavors to incorporate.
2. Season the salmon steaks with salt and pepper; grill them on both sides for 8 minutes in total. Serve the salmon steaks warm on a bed of the radish salad.

NUTRITION VALUES: Calories: 338, Fat: 21.7g, Net Carbs: 3.1g, Protein: 28.5g

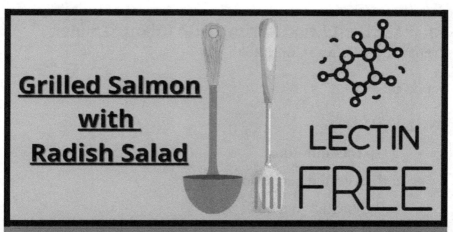

Grilled Salmon with Radish Salad

LECTIN FREE

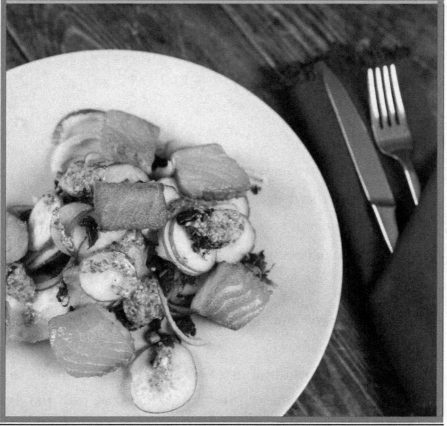

33. **Coconut Fried Shrimp with Cilantro Sauce**
Preparation Time: 15 minutes

Servings: 2

INGREDIENTS

- 2 tsp coconut flour
- 2 tbsp grated pecorino cheese
- 1 egg, beaten in a bowl
- ¼ tsp curry powder
- ½ pound shrimp, shelled
- 3 tbsp coconut oil
- Salt to taste
- Sauce
- 2 tbsp ghee
- 2 tbsp cilantro leaves, chopped
- ½ onion, diced
- ½ cup coconut cream
- ½ ounce paneer cheese, grated

DIRECTIONS

1. Combine coconut flour, pecorino cheese, curry powder, and salt in a bowl.
2. Melt the coconut oil in a skillet over medium heat. Dip the shrimp in the egg first, and then coat with the dry mixture. Fry until golden and crispy, about 5 minutes.

3. In another skillet, melt the ghee. Add onion and cook for 3 minutes. Add curry and cilantro and cook for 30 seconds. Stir in coconut cream and paneer cheese and cook until thickened. Add the shrimp and coat well. Serve warm.

NUTRITION VALUES: Calories: 741, Fat: 64g, Net Carbs: 4.3g, Protein: 34.4g

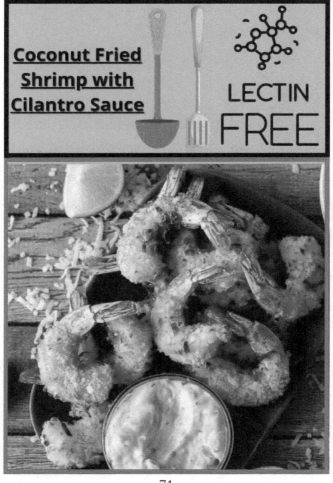

34. Catalan Shrimp with Garlic

Preparation Time: 22 minutes

Servings: 2-4

INGREDIENTS

- ¼ cup olive oil, divided
- 1 pound shrimp, peeled and deveined
- Salt to taste
- ¼ tsp cayenne pepper
- 3 garlic cloves, sliced
- 2 tbsp chopped parsley

DIRECTIONS

1. Warm olive oil in a large skillet over medium heat. Reduce the heat and add the garlic; cook for 6-8 minutes, but make sure it doesn't brown or burn. Add the shrimp, season with salt and cayenne pepper, stir for one minute and turn off the heat. Let the shrimp finish cooking with the heat of the hot oil for about 8-10 minutes. Serve garnished with parsley.

NUTRITION VALUES: Calories: 441, Fat: 29g, Net Carbs: 1.2g, Protein: 43g

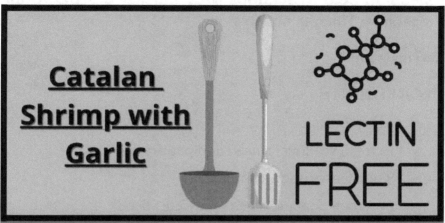

Catalan Shrimp with Garlic

LECTIN FREE

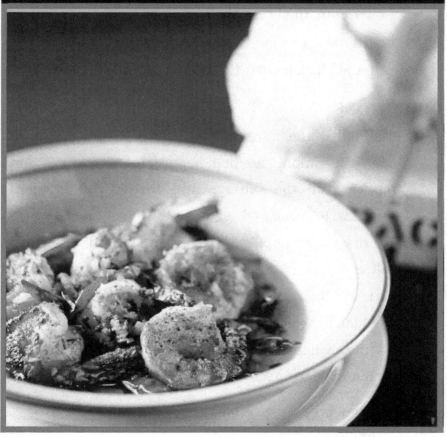

35.   Pan-Seared Scallops with Sausage & Mozzarella

Preparation Time: 15 minutes

Servings: 2-4

INGREDIENTS

- 2 tbsp butter
- 12 fresh scallops, rinsed and pat dry
- 8 ounces sausage, chopped
- 1 red bell pepper, seeds removed, sliced
- 1 red onion, finely chopped
- 1 cup Grana Padano cheese, grated
- Salt and black pepper to taste

DIRECTIONS

1. Melt half of the butter in a skillet over medium heat, and cook the onion and bell pepper for 5 minutes until tender. Add the sausage and stir-fry for another 5 minutes. Remove and set aside.
2. Pat dry the scallops with paper towels, and season with salt and pepper. Add the remaining butter to the skillet and sear the scallops for 2 minutes on each side to have a golden brown color. Add the sausage mixture back and warm through. Transfer to serving platter and top with Grana Padano cheese.

NUTRITION VALUES: Calories: 834, Fat: 62g, Net Carbs: 9,5g, Protein: 56g

36. Round Zucchini Stuffed with Shrimp and Tomato

Preparation Time: 35 minutes

Servings: 2

INGREDIENTS

- 1 pound zucchinis, tops removed and reserved
- 1 lb small shrimp, peeled, deveined
- ¼ onion, chopped
- 1 tsp olive oil
- 1 small tomato, chopped
- Salt and black pepper to taste
- 1 tbsp basil leaves, chopped

DIRECTIONS

1. Scoop out the seeds of the zucchinis with a spoon and set aside.
2. Warm olive oil in a skillet and sauté the onion and tomato for 3 minutes. Add the shrimp, zucchini flesh, basil leaves, salt, and pepper and cook for another 5 minutes.
3. Fill the zucchini shells with the mixture. Cover with the zucchini tops and place them on a greased baking sheet to cook for 15 to 20 minutes at 390 F. The shrimp should no longer be pink by this time. Remove the zucchinis and serve with tomato and mozzarella salad.

NUTRITION VALUES: Calories: 252, Fat: 6.4g, Net Carbs: 8.9g, Protein: 37.6g

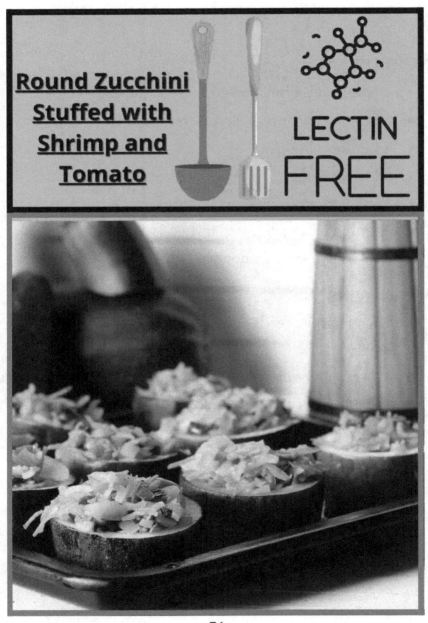

Round Zucchini Stuffed with Shrimp and Tomato

LECTIN FREE

37.   **Mustardy Crab Cakes**
Preparation Time: 15 minutes

Servings: 2-4

INGREDIENTS

- 1 tbsp coconut oil
- 1 pound lump crab meat
- 1 tsp Dijon mustard
- 1 egg
- ¼ cup mayonnaise
- 1 tbsp coconut flour
- 1 tbsp cilantro, chopped

DIRECTIONS

1. In a bowl, add crab meat, mustard, mayonnaise, coconut flour, egg, cilantro, salt, and black pepper; mix well to combine. Make patties out of the mixture.
2. Melt the coconut oil in a skillet over medium heat. Add the crab patties and cook for about 2-3 minutes per side. Remove with a perforated spoon and drain on kitchen paper.

NUTRITION VALUES: Calories: 315, Fat: 24.5g, Net Carbs: 1.6g, Protein: 15.3g

38.   Chimichurri Tiger Shrimp

Preparation Time: 55 minutes

Servings: 2-4

INGREDIENTS

- 1 pound tiger shrimp, peeled and deveined
- 2 tbsp olive oil
- 1 garlic clove, minced
- Juice of 1 lime
- Salt and black pepper to taste
- Chimichurri
- Salt and black pepper to taste
- ¼ cup extra-virgin olive oil
- 2 garlic cloves, minced
- 1 lime, juiced
- ¼ cup red wine vinegar
- 2 cups parsley, minced
- ¼ tsp red pepper flakes

DIRECTIONS

1. Combine the shrimp, olive oil, garlic, and lime juice, in a bowl, and let marinate in the fridge for 30 minutes.
2. To make the chimichurri dressing, blitz the chimichurri ingredients in a blender until smooth; set aside. Preheat your grill to medium. Add shrimp and cook about 2 minutes per side.

3. Serve shrimp drizzled with the chimichurri dressing.

NUTRITION VALUES: Calories: 523, Fat: 30.3g, Net Carbs: 7.2g, Protein: 49g

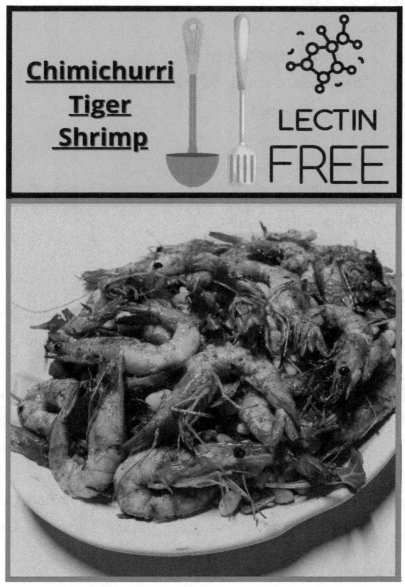

39. **Mussel Coconut Curry**

Preparation Time: 25 minutes

Servings: 2-4

INGREDIENTS

- 2 tbsp cup coconut oil
- 2 green onions, chopped
- 1 lb mussels, cleaned, de-bearded
- 1 shallot, chopped
- 1 garlic clove, minced
- ½ cup coconut milk
- ½ cup white wine
- 1 tsp red curry powder
- 2 tbsp parsley, chopped

DIRECTIONS

1. Cook the shallots and garlic in the wine over low heat. Stir in the coconut milk and red curry powder and cook for 3 minutes.
2. Add the mussels and steam for 7 minutes or until their shells are opened. Then, use a slotted spoon to remove to a bowl leaving the sauce in the pan. Discard any closed mussels at this point.
3. Stir the coconut oil into the sauce, turn the heat off, and stir in the parsley and green onions. Serve the sauce immediately with a butternut squash mash.

NUTRITION VALUES: Calories: 356, Fat: 20.6g, Net Carbs: 0.3g, Protein: 21.1g

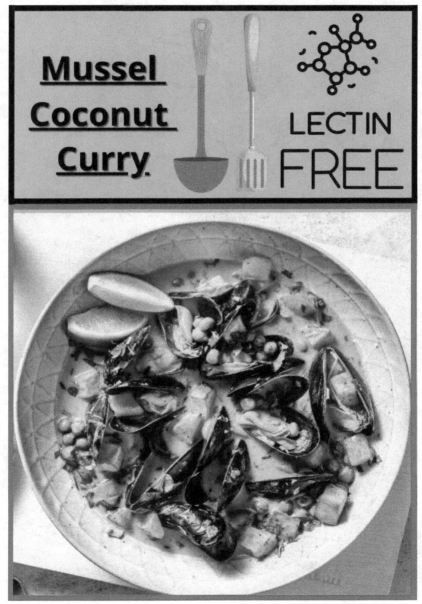

POULTRY

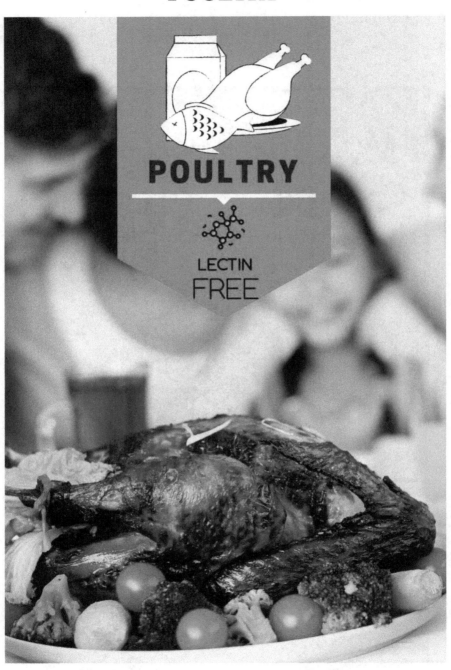

40. **Turkey And Tomato Curry**

Preparation Time: 30 minutes

Servings: 4

INGREDIENTS

- 20 ounces canned tomatoes; chopped.
- 18 ounces turkey meat; minced
- 1 tablespoons turmeric
- 1 tablespoon cumin; ground
- 1 tablespoon coriander; ground
- 3 ounces spinach
- 2 tablespoons coconut oil
- 2 tablespoons coconut cream
- 2 garlic cloves; minced
- 2 yellow onions; sliced
- 2 tablespoons ginger; grated
- 2 tablespoons chili powder
- Salt and black pepper to the taste.

DIRECTIONS

1. Heat up a pan with the coconut oil over medium heat; add onion; stir and cook for 5 minutes
2. Add ginger and garlic; stir and cook for 1 minute
3. Add tomatoes, salt, pepper, coriander, cumin, turmeric and chili powder and stir.
4. Add coconut cream; stir and cook for 10 minutes

5. Blend using an immersion blender and mix with spinach and turkey meat.

6. Bring to a simmer, cook for 15 minutes more and serve

NUTRITION VALUES: Calories: 240; Fat 4; Fiber : 3; Carbs 2; Protein 12

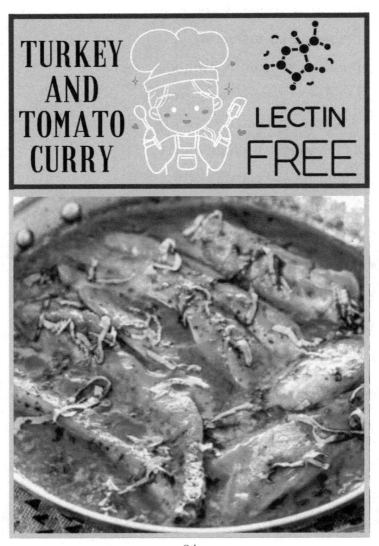

41. Skillet Chicken And Mushrooms

Preparation Time: 40 minutes

Servings: 4

INGREDIENTS

- 4 chicken thighs
- 2 cups mushrooms; sliced
- 1/2 teaspoon onion powder
- 1/4 cup ghee
- 1/2 teaspoon garlic powder
- 1/2 cup water
- 1 teaspoon Dijon mustard
- 1 tablespoon tarragon; chopped.
- Salt and black pepper to the taste.

DIRECTIONS

1. Heat up a pan with half of the ghee over medium high heat; add chicken thighs, season them with salt, pepper, garlic powder and onion powder, cook the for 3 minutes on each side and transfer to a bowl.
2. Heat up the same pan with the rest of the ghee over medium high heat; add mushrooms; stir and cook for 5 minutes
3. Add mustard and water and stir well.
4. Return chicken pieces to the pan; stir, cover and cook for 15 minutes

5. Add tarragon; stir, cook for 5 minutes, divide between plates and serve

NUTRITION VALUES: Calories: 453; Fat 32; Fiber 6; Carbs 1; Protein 36

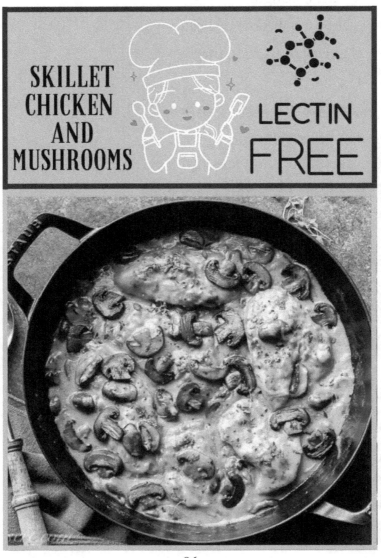

42.   **<u>Turkey Soup Recipe</u>**

Preparation Time: 40 minutes

Servings: 4

INGREDIENTS

- 3 cups turkey; cooked and shredded
- 3 celery stalks; chopped.
- 1 yellow onion; chopped.
- 1 tablespoon ghee
- 6 cups turkey stock
- 3 cups baked spaghetti squash; chopped.
- 1/4 cup parsley; chopped.
- Salt and black pepper to the taste.

DIRECTIONS

1. Heat up a pot with the ghee over medium high heat; add celery and onion; stir and cook for 5 minutes
2. Add parsley, stock, turkey meat, salt and pepper; stir and cook for 20 minutes
3. Add spaghetti squash; stir and cook turkey soup for 10 minutes more
4. Divide into bowls and serve

NUTRITION VALUES: Calories: 150; Fat 4; Fiber 1; Carbs 3; Protein 10

43. <u>**Duck Breast With Tasty Veggies**</u>

Preparation Time: 20 minutes

Servings: 2

INGREDIENTS

- 2 duck breasts; skin on and thinly sliced
- 2 zucchinis; sliced
- 1 spring onion stack; chopped.
- 1 daikon; chopped.
- 2 green bell peppers; chopped.
- 1 tablespoon coconut oil
- Salt and black pepper to the taste.

DIRECTIONS

1. Heat up a pan with the oil over medium high heat; add spring onions; stir and cook for 2 minutes
2. Add zucchinis, daikon, bell peppers, salt and pepper; stir and cook for 10 minutes more
3. Heat up another pan over medium high heat; add duck slices, cook for 3 minutes on each side and transfer to the pan with the veggies
4. Cook everything for 3 minutes more, divide between plates and serve

NUTRITION VALUES: Calories: 450; Fat 23; Fiber 3; Carbs 8; Protein 50

44. **Italian Chicken**

Preparation Time: 1 hour 10 minutes

Servings: 6

INGREDIENTS

- 4 chicken thighs
- 8 ounces mushrooms; chopped.
- 1 pound Italian sausage; chopped.
- 2 tablespoons avocado oil
- 6 cherry peppers; chopped.
- 1 red bell pepper; chopped.
- 1 red onion; sliced
- 1/2 cup chicken stock
- 2 tablespoons garlic; minced
- 2 cups cherry tomatoes; halved
- 1 tablespoon balsamic vinegar
- 2 teaspoons oregano; dried
- Some chopped parsley for serving
- Salt and black pepper to the taste.

DIRECTIONS

1. Heat up a pan with half of the oil over medium heat; add sausages; stir, brown for a few minutes and transfer to a plate
2. Heat up the pan again with the rest of the oil over medium heat; add chicken thighs, season with salt and

pepper, cook for 3 minutes on each side and transfer to a plate

3. Heat up the pan again over medium heat; add cherry peppers, mushrooms, onion and bell pepper; stir and cook for 4 minutes

4. Add garlic; stir and cook for 2 minutes

5. Add stock, vinegar, salt, pepper, oregano and cherry tomatoes and stir.

6. Add chicken pieces and sausages ones; stir gently, transfer everything to the oven at 400 degrees and bake for 30 minutes

7. Sprinkle parsley, divide between plates and serve

NUTRITION VALUES: Calories: 340; Fat 33; Fiber 3; Carbs 4; Protein 20

45. __Tasty Turkey Pie__

Preparation Time: 50 minutes

Servings: 6

INGREDIENTS

- 2 cups turkey stock
- 1 cup turkey meat; cooked and shredded
- 1/2 cup kale; chopped.
- 1 teaspoon thyme; chopped.
- 1/4 teaspoon paprika
- 1/2 cup butternut squash; peeled and chopped.
- 1/2 cup cheddar cheese; shredded
- 1/4 teaspoon garlic powder
- 1/4 teaspoon xanthan gum
- Cooking spray
- Salt and black pepper to the taste.

For the crust:

- 1/4 cup ghee
- 1/4 teaspoon xanthan gum
- 1/4 cup cheddar cheese
- 2 cups almond flour
- A pinch of salt
- 1 egg

DIRECTIONS

1. Heat up a pot with the stock over medium heat.

2. Add squash and turkey meat; stir and cook for 10 minutes
3. Add garlic powder, kale, thyme, paprika, salt, pepper and 1/2 cup cheddar cheese and stir well.
4. In a bowl, mix 1/4 teaspoon xanthan gum with 1/2 cup stock from the pot; stir well and add everything to the pot.
5. Take off heat and then leave aside for now.
6. In a bowl, mix flour with 1/4 teaspoon xanthan gum and a pinch of salt and stir.
7. Add ghee, egg and 1/4 cup cheddar cheese and stir everything until you obtain your pie crust dough.
8. Shape a ball and keep in the fridge for now.
9. Spray a baking dish with cooking spray and spread pie filling on the bottom.
10. Transfer dough to a working surface, roll into a circle and top filling with this
11. Press well and seal edges, introduce in the oven at 350 degrees F and bake for 35 minutes
12. Leave the pie to cool down a bit and serve

NUTRITION VALUES: Calories: 320; Fat 23; Fiber 8; Carbs 6; Protein 16

46. **Baked Chicken**

Preparation Time: 30 minutes

Servings: 4

INGREDIENTS

- 4 chicken breasts
- 4 bacon strips
- 3 green onions; chopped.
- 4 ounces ranch dressing
- 1 ounce coconut aminos
- 4 ounces cheddar cheese; grated
- 2 tablespoons coconut oil

DIRECTIONS

1. Heat up a pan with the oil over high heat; add chicken breasts, cook for 7 minutes, flip and cook for 7 more minutes
2. Meanwhile; heat up another pan over medium high heat; add bacon, cook until it's crispy, transfer to paper towels, drain grease and crumble
3. Transfer chicken breast to a baking dish, add coconut aminos, crumbled bacon, cheese and green onions on top, introduce in your oven, set on broiler and cook at a high temperature for 5 minutes more
4. Divide between plates and serve hot.

NUTRITION VALUES: Calories: 450; Fat 24; Fiber 0; Carbs 3; Protein 60

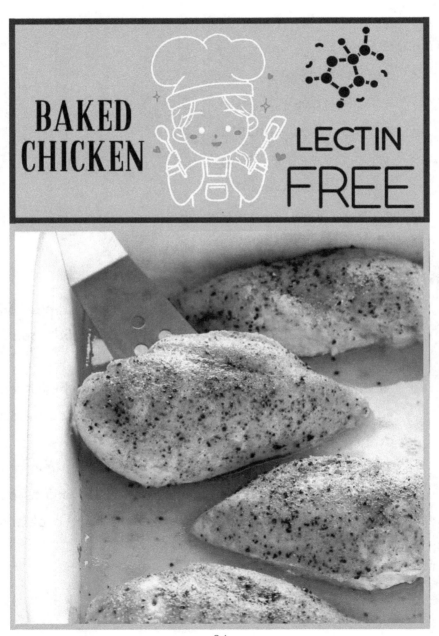

47. **Creamy Chicken Soup Recipe**

Preparation Time: 30 minutes

Servings: 4

INGREDIENTS

- 2 cups chicken meat; cooked and shredded
- 3 tablespoons ghee
- 1/4 cup celery; chopped.
- 1/2 cup sour cream
- 1/3 cup red sauce
- 4 cups chicken stock
- 4 ounces cream cheese
- Salt and black pepper to the taste.

DIRECTIONS

1. In your blender, mix stock with red sauce, cream cheese, ghee, salt, pepper and sour cream and pulse well.
2. Transfer this to a pot, heat up over medium heat and add celery and chicken.
3. Stir, simmer for a few minutes, divide into bowls and serve

NUTRITION VALUES: Calories: 400; Fat 23; Fiber 5; Carbs 5; Protein 30

48. Chicken And Olives Tapenade

Preparation Time: 20 minutes

Servings: 2

INGREDIENTS

- 1 chicken breast cut into 4 pieces
- 1/2 cup olives tapenade
- 3 garlic cloves; crushed.
- 2 tablespoons coconut oil

For the tapenade:

- 1 cup black olives; pitted
- 1/4 cup parsley; chopped.
- 2 tablespoons olive oil
- Salt and black pepper to the taste.
- 1 tablespoons lemon juice

DIRECTIONS

1. In your food processor, mix olives with salt, pepper, 2 tablespoons olive oil, lemon juice and parsley, blend very well and transfer to a bowl.
2. Heat up a pan with the coconut oil over medium heat; add garlic; stir and cook for 2 minutes
3. Add chicken pieces and cook for 4 minutes on each side
4. Divide chicken on plates and top with the olives tapenade

NUTRITION VALUES: Calories: 130; Fat 12; Fiber 0; Carbs 3; Protein 20

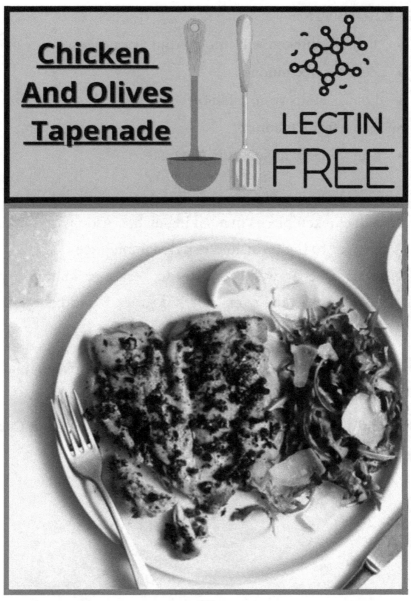

49.   Lemon Chicken

Preparation Time: 55 minutes

Servings: 6

INGREDIENTS

- 1 whole chicken; cut into medium pieces
- Zest from 2 lemons
- Lemon rinds from 2 lemons
- Juice from 2 lemons
- Salt and black pepper to the taste.

DIRECTIONS

1. Put chicken pieces in a baking dish, season with salt and pepper to the taste. and drizzle lemon juice
2. Toss to coat well, add lemon zest and lemon rinds, introduce in the oven at 375 degrees F and bake for 45 minutes

3. Discard lemon rinds, divide chicken between plates, drizzle sauce from the baking dish over it and serve

NUTRITION VALUES: Calories: 334; Fat 24; Fiber 2; Carbs
4. 5; Protein 27

Lemon Chicken

LECTIN
FREE

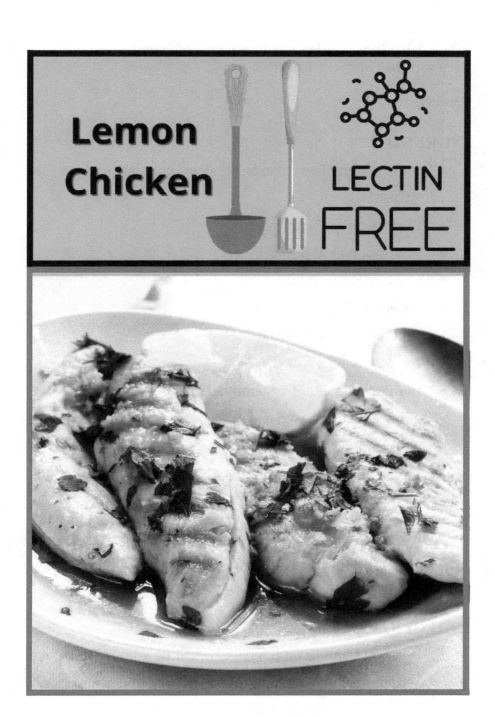

50. **Chicken Fajitas**

Preparation Time: 25 minutes

Servings: 4

INGREDIENTS

- 2 pounds chicken breasts; skinless, boneless and cut into strips
- 1 teaspoon garlic powder
- 1 teaspoon chili powder
- 2 teaspoons cumin
- 1 green bell pepper; sliced
- 1 red bell pepper; sliced
- 1 yellow onion; sliced
- 1 tablespoon cilantro; chopped.
- 2 limes; cut into wedges
- 2 tablespoons lime juice
- 1 teaspoon sweet paprika
- 2 tablespoons coconut oil
- 1 teaspoon coriander; ground
- 1 avocado; pitted, peeled and sliced
- Salt and black pepper to the taste.

DIRECTIONS

1. In a bowl, mix lime juice with chili powder, cumin, salt, pepper, garlic powder, paprika and coriander and stir.
2. Add chicken pieces and toss to coat well.

3. Heat up a pan with half of the oil over medium high heat; add chicken, cook for 3 minutes on each side and transfer to a bowl.

4. Heat up the pan with the rest of the oil over medium heat; add onion and all bell peppers; stir and cook for 6 minutes

5. Return chicken to pan, add more salt and pepper; stir and divide between plates

6. Top with avocado, lime wedges and cilantro and serve

NUTRITION VALUES: Calories: 240; Fat 10; Fiber 2; Carbs 5; Protein 20

51. Chicken And Green Onion Sauce Recipe

Preparation Time: 37 minutes

Servings: 4

INGREDIENTS

- 4 chicken breast halves; skinless and boneless
- 8 ounces sour cream
- 2 tablespoons ghee
- 1 green onion; chopped.
- Salt and black pepper to the taste.

DIRECTIONS

1. Heat up a pan with the ghee over medium high heat; add chicken pieces, season with salt and pepper, cover, reduce heat and simmer for 10 minutes
2. Uncover pan, turn chicken pieces and cook them covered for 10 minutes more
3. Add green onions; stir and cook for 2 minutes more
4. Take off heat; add more salt and pepper if needed, add sour cream; stir well, cover pan and leave aside for 5 minutes
5. Stir again, divide between plates and serve

NUTRITION VALUES: Calories: 200; Fat 7; Fiber 2; Carbs 1; Protein 8

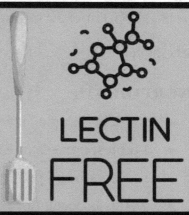

Chicken And Green Onion Sauce Recipe

LECTIN FREE

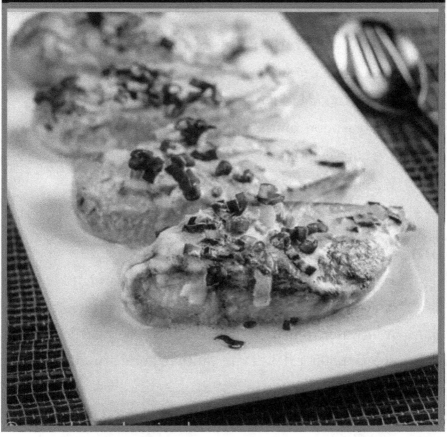

52. Chicken Stir Fry

Preparation Time: 22 minutes

Servings: 2

INGREDIENTS

- 2 chicken thighs; skinless, boneless cut into thin strips
- 1 tablespoon sesame oil
- 1 teaspoon red pepper flakes
- 2 cups broccoli florets
- 1/4 cup tamari sauce
- 1/2 teaspoon garlic powder
- 1 teaspoon onion powder
- 1 tablespoon ginger; grated
- 1/2 teaspoon xanthan gum
- 1/2 cup scallions; chopped.
- 1/2 cup water
- 1 tablespoon stevia

DIRECTIONS

1. Heat up a pan with the oil over medium high heat; add chicken and ginger; stir and cook for 3 minutes
2. Add water, tamari sauce, onion powder, garlic powder, stevia, pepper flakes and xanthan gum; stir and cook for 5 minutes
3. Add broccoli and scallions; stir, cook for 2 minutes more and divide between plates. Serve hot.

NUTRITION VALUES: Calories: 210; Fat 10; Fiber 3; Carbs 5; Protein 20

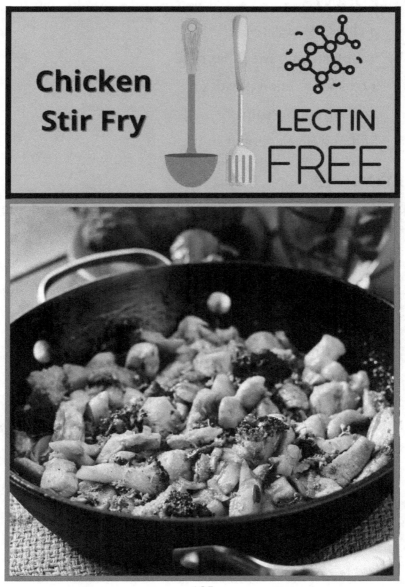

53. Chicken And Sour Cream Sauce

Preparation Time: 50 minutes

Servings: 4

INGREDIENTS

- 4 chicken thighs
- 2 tablespoons sweet paprika
- 1 teaspoon onion powder
- 1/4 cup sour cream
- Salt and black pepper to the taste.

DIRECTIONS

1. In a bowl, mix paprika with salt, pepper and onion powder and stir.
2. Season chicken pieces with this paprika mix, arrange them on a lined baking sheet and bake in the oven at 400 degrees F for 40 minutes
3. Divide chicken on plates and leave aside for now.
4. Pour juices from the pan into a bowl and add sour cream.
5. Stir this sauce very well and drizzle over chicken.

NUTRITION VALUES: Calories: 384; Fat 31; Fiber 2; Carbs 1; Protein 33

Chicken And Sour Cream Sauce

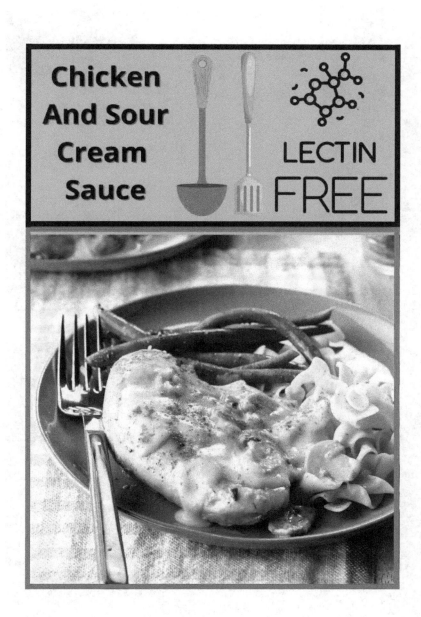

MEAT

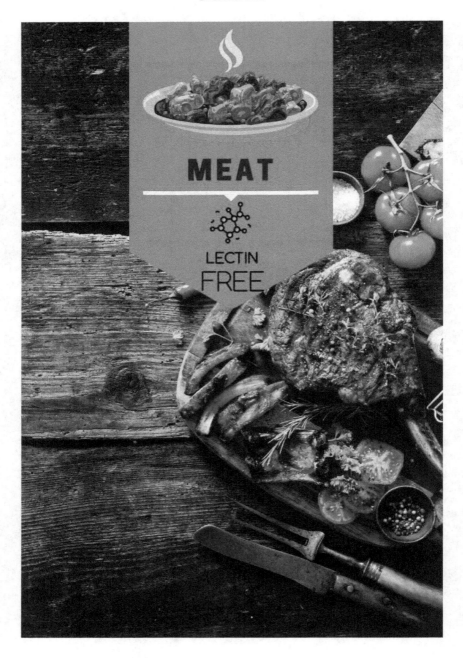

54. **Beef And Spinach**

Preparation Time: 22 minutes

Servings: 2

INGREDIENTS

- 1 big oyster mushroom; chopped
- 2 tbsp. almonds; chopped
- 2 tbsp. ghee
- 4 oz. beef; ground
- 1/2 tsp. chili flakes
- A pinch of sea salt
- White pepper to the taste
- 1 tbsp. capers
- 1/4 cup kalamata olives; pitted
- 1 tbsp. roasted almond butter
- 3 oz. spinach leaves; torn

DIRECTIONS

1. Heat up a pan with the ghee over medium high heat, add mushroom, stir and cook for 3 minutes.
2. Add almonds, stir and cook for 1 minute. Add beef, chili flakes, a pinch of salt and white pepper, stir and cook for 6 minutes.
3. Add almond butter, capers, olives and spinach, stir; cook for a couple more minutes, divide into 2 bowls and serve.

NUTRITION VALUES: Calories: 320; Fat: 2g; Fiber: 5g; Carbs: 9g; Protein: 23g

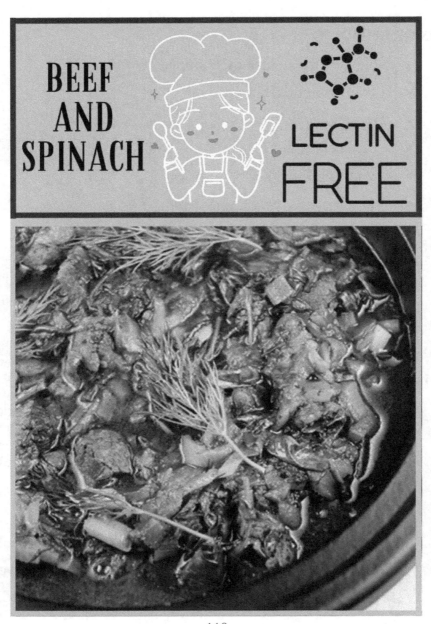

55. Lavender Lamb Chops

Preparation Time: 2 hours 10 minutes

Servings: 4

INGREDIENTS

- 4 lamb chops
- 2 garlic cloves; minced
- 1 tbsp. lavender; chopped
- 2 tbsp. rosemary; chopped
- A pinch of sea salt
- Black pepper to the taste
- 1 tbsp. ghee
- 3 small orange peel; grated

DIRECTIONS

1. In a bowl; mix lamb chops with garlic, lavender, rosemary, orange peel, a pinch of salt and black pepper, rub well and keep in the fridge for 2 hours.
2. Heat up your grill over medium high heat, grease it with the ghee, place lamb chops on it, grill for 5 minutes on each side, divide between plates and serve with a side salad on the side.

NUTRITION VALUES: Calories: 160; Fat: 2g; Fiber: 1g; Carbs: 4g; Protein: 10g

56.   Beef Patties

Preparation Time: 35 minutes

Servings: 4

INGREDIENTS

- 2 sweet potatoes; boiled and grated
- 1 lb. beef; ground
- 1 cup red onion; chopped
- 2 Serrano peppers; chopped
- 1 small ginger piece; grated
- A handful cilantro; chopped
- 4 garlic cloves; minced
- 1/2 tsp. meat masala
- A pinch of cayenne pepper
- 1/4 tsp. turmeric powder
- Black pepper to the taste
- 1 egg; whisked
- 4 tbsp. almond meal
- 1 cup water
- 5 tbsp. ghee

DIRECTIONS

1. Heat up a pan over medium high heat, add beef, masala, turmeric, black pepper to the taste and cayenne pepper, stir and brown for a few minutes.

2. Add water, stir; cook for 10 minutes more and take off heat.
3. Heat up a pan with 2 tbsp. ghee over medium heat, add Serrano peppers and onion, stir and cook for 2 minutes.
4. Add garlic and ginger, stir and cook for 1 minute more.
5. Add cilantro and the meat mixture, stir well and take off heat.
6. Add grated sweet potatoes, stir well, cool everything down and shape patties from this mix.
7. Put the egg in a bowl and almond meal in another.
8. Dip patties in egg and then in almond meal.
9. Heat up a pan with the rest of the ghee over medium heat, add beef patties, cook them well on one side, flip, cook on the other as well and transfer them to paper towels. Serve them with a side salad.

NUTRITION VALUES: Calories: 180; Fat: 3g; Fiber: 3g; Carbs: 6g; Protein: 15g

57. Thai Lamb Chops

Preparation Time: 1 hour 15 minutes

Servings: 4

INGREDIENTS

- 1/3 cup basil; chopped
- 2 garlic cloves; chopped
- 2 tbsp. Thai green curry paste
- 2 tbsp. avocado oil
- 1 tbsp. gluten free tamari sauce
- 1 small ginger piece; grated
- 2 lbs. lamb chops
- 1 tbsp. coconut oil
- 1 tbsp. coconut aminos

DIRECTIONS

1. In your food processor, mix basil with garlic, curry paste, avocado oil, tamari sauce, aminos and ginger and blend really well.
2. Put lamb chops in a bowl; add basil mix over them, toss well and keep in the fridge for 1 hour.
3. Heat up a pan with the coconut oil over medium high heat, add lamb chops, cook for 2 minutes on each side, introduce pan in the oven and roast lamb at 400 °F for 10 minutes. Serve lamb chops with a side salad.

NUTRITION VALUES: Calories: 170; Fat: 3g; Fiber: 2g; Carbs: 5g; Protein: 14g

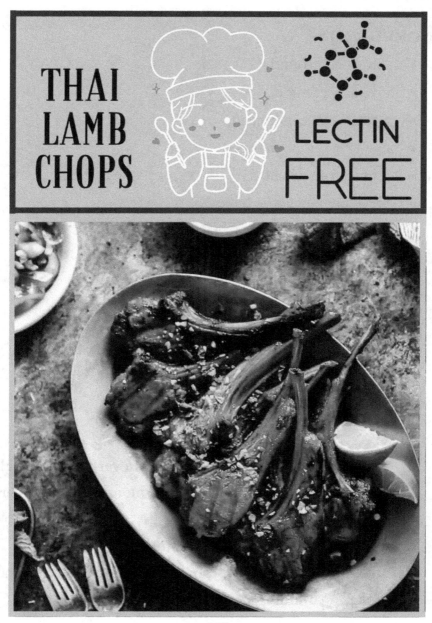

58.   Greek Beef Bowls

Preparation Time: 35 minutes

Servings: 4

INGREDIENTS

- 1 lb. beef; ground
- 1 tbsp. coconut oil
- 2 garlic cloves; minced
- 1 yellow onion; chopped
- A pinch of sea salt
- Black pepper to the taste
- 1 tbsp. savory; dried
- 1 tbsp. parsley; dried
- 2 tbsp. oregano; dried
- 3 oz. kale; chopped
- 3 oz. endives; chopped
- 1/4 cup kalamata olives; pitted and sliced
- 1/4 cup green olives; pitted and sliced

DIRECTIONS

1. Heat up a pan with the coconut oil over medium high heat, add garlic, onion, a pinch of salt and black pepper, stir and cook for 3 minutes.
2. Add beef, stir and cook for 10 minutes.
3. Add endives, kale, savory, oregano and parsley, stir and cook for 5 minutes more.

4. Add green and kalamata olives, stir; place in preheated broiler and broil for 4 minutes. Divide into bowls and serve.

NUTRITION VALUES: Calories: 367; Fat: 7g; Fiber: 4g; Carbs: 9g; Protein: 30g

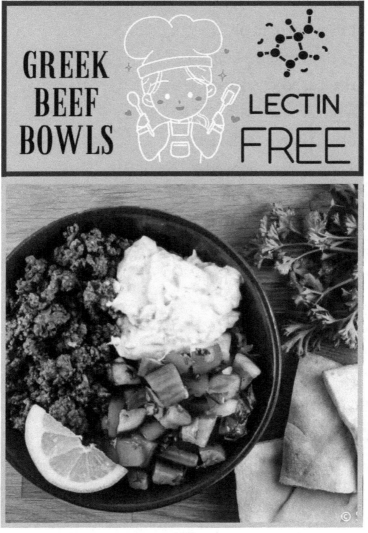

59. Beef And Basil

Preparation Time: 26 minutes

Servings: 4

INGREDIENTS

- 6 garlic cloves; minced
- 2 red chilies; chopped
- 1 tbsp. coconut oil
- 1 yellow onion; chopped
- 1½ lbs. beef; ground
- A pinch of sea salt
- Black pepper to the taste
- 3 cups basil; chopped
- 1/2 cup chicken stock
- 2 cups carrot; grated
- 4 tbsp. lime juice
- 2 tbsp. coconut aminos
- 1 tbsp. olive oil
- 1/2 tbsp. honey
- Cauliflower rice for serving

DIRECTIONS

1. Heat up a pan with the coconut oil over medium heat, add onions and a pinch of salt, stir and cook for 4 minutes.

2. Add garlic and chili peppers, stir and cook for 1 minute more.

3. Add beef and black pepper, stir and brown everything for 8 minutes. Add stock and half of the basil, stir and cook for 2 minutes more.

4. In a bowl; mix carrots with 1 tbsp. lime juice, the rest of the basil and the olive oil and stir well.

5. In another bowl; mix coconut aminos with the rest of the lime juice and honey and also stir very well.

6. Divide cauliflower rice on plates,add beef and carrot mix on top and drizzle the honey sauce you've made at the end.

NUTRITION VALUES: Calories: 200; Fat: 3g; Fiber: 5g; Carbs: 7g; Protein: 17g

60. **Hamburger Salad**

Preparation Time: 18 minutes

Servings: 4

INGREDIENTS

- 2 garlic cloves; minced
- 1 sweet onion; chopped
- 1 tbsp. coconut oil
- 1 lb. beef; ground
- 1 cup cherry tomatoes; chopped
- 1 dill pickle; chopped
- 1 lettuce head; leaves separated and chopped
- A pinch of sea salt
- Black pepper to the taste

For the dressing:

- 2 tbsp. water
- 4 tbsp. mayonnaise
- 2 tbsp. Paleo ketchup
- 1 tbsp. yellow onion; chopped
- 1 tsp. balsamic vinegar
- 1 tbsp. pickle; minced

DIRECTIONS

1. Heat up a pan with the oil over medium heat, add garlic and onion, stir and cook for 2 minutes.

2. Add beef, a pinch of sea salt and black pepper, stir; cook for 8 minutes more and take off heat.
3. In a salad bowl; combine beef mix and with lettuce leaves, 1 dill pickle and cherry tomatoes.
4. In another bowl; mix water with mayo, ketchup, yellow onion, vinegar and 1 tbsp. pickle and whisk well. Drizzle this over salad, toss to coat and serve.

NUTRITION VALUES: Calories: 170; Fat: 3g; Fiber: 2g; Carbs: 5g; Protein: 12g

61. Lamb Chops

Preparation Time: 20 minutes

Servings: 6

INGREDIENTS

- 3 tbsp. coconut aminos
- 4 tbsp. olive oil
- 2 tbsp. ginger; grated
- 8 lamb chops
- 1 tbsp. parsley; chopped
- 2 garlic cloves; minced
- A pinch of sea salt
- Black pepper to the taste

DIRECTIONS

1. In a bowl; mix oil with aminos, parsley, ginger and garlic and stir well.
2. Place lamb chops on a preheated grill over medium high heat, season them with a pinch of salt and black pepper to the taste and grill them for 4 minutes on each side basting them with the oil and ginger mix you've made. Leave lamb chops to cool down for a couple of minutes and then serve.

NUTRITION VALUES: Calories: 160; Fat: 5g; Fiber: 0g; Carbs: 1g; Protein: 20g

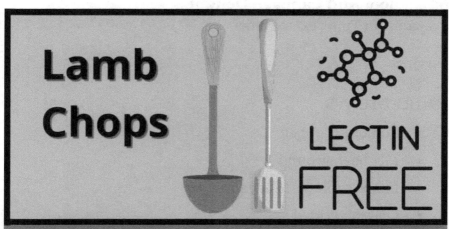

Lamb Chops

LECTIN FREE

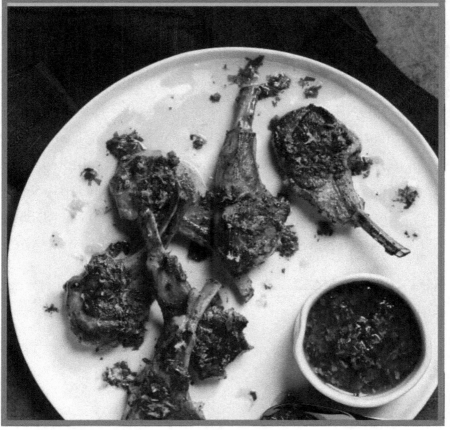

62.   **<u>Beef And Cabbage Delight</u>**

Preparation Time: 20 minutes

Servings: 4

INGREDIENTS

- 1 onion; chopped
- 1 lb. beef; ground
- 1 napa cabbage head; shredded
- 1 carrot; grated
- A pinch of sea salt
- Black pepper to the taste
- 2 tbsp. coconut oil

DIRECTIONS

1. Heat up a pan with the oil over medium high heat, add onion and beef, stir and brown them for 5 minutes.
2. Add carrots, cabbage, a pinch of salt and black pepper to the taste, stir and cook for 5 minutes more. Divide between plates and serve.

NUTRITION VALUES: Calories: 150; Fat: 1g; Fiber: 2g; Carbs: 5g; Protein: 9g

Beef And Cabbage Delight

LECTIN FREE

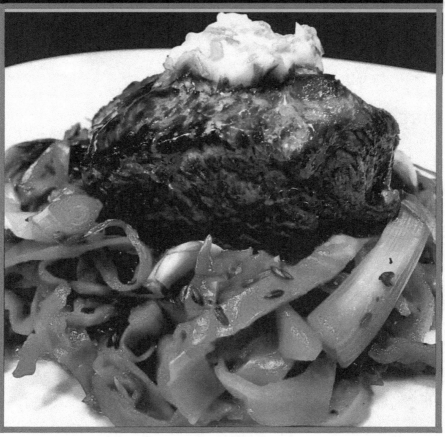

63. Slow Cooked Lamb Shanks

Preparation Time: 4 hours 10 minutes

Servings: 4

INGREDIENTS

- 2 big lamb shanks
- A pinch of sea salt
- 1 garlic head; cloves peeled
- 4 tbsp. olive oil
- Juice of 1/2 lemon
- Zest from 1/2 lemon; grated
- 1/2 tsp. oregano; dried

DIRECTIONS

1. Put lamb shanks in your slow cooker, sprinkle a pinch of sea salt, add garlic cloves, cover and cook on High for 4 hours.
2. In a bowl; mix olive oil with lemon juice, lemon zest and oregano and whisk well.
3. Transfer lamb shanks to a cutting board, discard bones, shred meat and divide between plates. Drizzle the lemon dressing on top and serve with a Paleo side salad.

NUTRITION VALUES: Calories: 180; Fat: 2g; Fiber: 2g; Carbs: 4g; Protein: 9g

64. **Rosemary Lamb Chops**
Preparation Time: 20 minutes

Servings: 4

INGREDIENTS
- 4 lamb chops
- 12 rosemary springs
- 4 garlic cloves; halved
- 1/2 tsp. black peppercorns
- 3 tbsp. avocado oil
- A pinch of sea salt

DIRECTIONS
1. In a bowl; mix lamb chops with a pinch of salt, black peppercorns and oil and massage well.
2. Spread lamb chops on a lined baking sheet and add garlic next to them. Rub rosemary into your palms and add over lamb chops.
3. Introduce everything in preheated broiler over medium high heat for 10 minutes, divide between plates and serve.

NUTRITION VALUES: Calories: 160; Fat: 3g; Fiber: 1g; Carbs: 2g; Protein: 20g

65. **Slow-Cooked Beef**
Preparation Time: 8 hours 50 minutes

Servings: 4

INGREDIENTS

- 2 cups beef stock
- 1/4 cup honey
- 1 cup tomato paste
- 1 cup balsamic vinegar
- 4 lbs. beef chuck
- 1 tbsp. mustard
- 1 tbsp. sweet paprika
- 1 tsp. onion powder
- 2 tbsp. chili powder
- 2 garlic cloves; minced
- Black pepper to the taste

DIRECTIONS

1. In a bowl; mix beef chuck with chili powder, paprika, onion powder, garlic and black pepper and rub well.
2. Transfer beef roast to your slow cooker, add stock over it, cover and cook on Low for 8 hours.
3. Meanwhile; heat up a pan over medium heat, add tomato paste, vinegar, mustard, honey and black pepper, stir; bring to a boil and cook for 12 minutes.
4. Transfer beef roast to a cutting board, leave it to cool down a bit, shred with a fork and return to your crock pot.

5. Add the sauce you've made in the pan, cover and cook everything on High for 30 minutes more. Divide this whole mix between plates and serve.

NUTRITION VALUES: Calories: 340; Fat: 5g; Fiber: 2g; Carbs: 5g; Protein: 24g

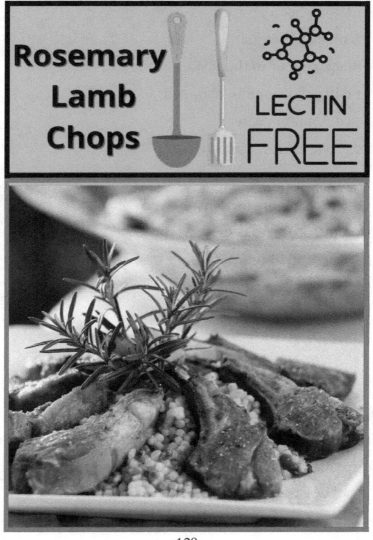

66. Lamb And Eggplant Puree

Preparation Time: 3 hours 25 minutes

Servings: 4

INGREDIENTS

- 4 lamb shoulder chops
- 1 tbsp. ghee
- A pinch of sea salt
- Black pepper to the taste
- 1 cup yellow onion; chopped
- 7 oz. tomato paste
- 2 garlic cloves; minced
- 3 cups water
- 8 oz. white mushrooms; halved

For the eggplant puree:

- Juice of 1 lemon
- 1/4 tsp. white pepper
- 2 eggplants
- 4 tbsp. ghee
- A pinch of sea salt

DIRECTIONS

1. Place eggplants on your preheated grill, cook for 30 minutes, flipping them from time to time, leave them to cool down and peel.

2. In your food processor, mix eggplant flesh with a pinch of salt, white pepper, lemon juice and 4 tbsp. ghee and pulse really well.

3. Spoon eggplant puree on plates and leave aside for now.

4. Heat up a pot with 1 tbsp. ghee, add lamb chops, season with a pinch of salt and black pepper to the taste, stir; brown them for a few minutes on each side and transfer to a plate.

5. Heat up the pot again over medium high heat, add onion, stir and cook for a couple of minutes.

6. Add garlic, stir and cook for 1 minute more.

7. Add mushrooms and tomato paste, stir and cook for 3 minutes more.

8. Add water, return lamb chops, stir; bring to a simmer, cover pot, reduce heat to medium-low heat and cook everything for 2 hours and 20 minutes. Divide lamb chops on eggplant puree and serve.

NUTRITION VALUES: Calories: 200; Fat: 3g; Fiber: 3g; Carbs: 5g; Protein: 10g

VEGETABLES

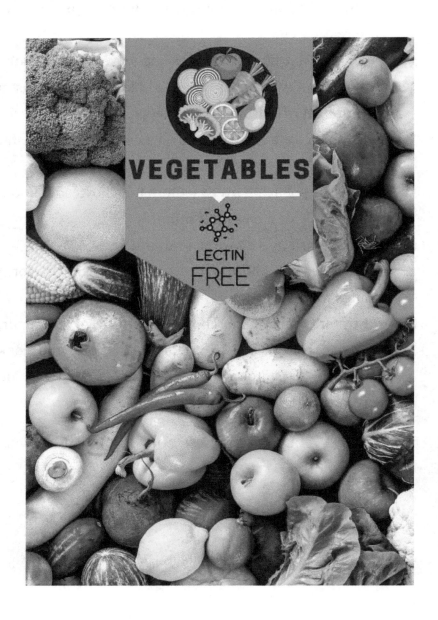

67. **Coconut Celery Soup**

Servings: 4

Preparation time: 10 minutes

Cooking time: 30 minutes

INGREDIENTS

- 6 cups celery stalk, chopped
- 2 cups vegetable stock
- 1 onion, chopped
- 1/2 tsp dill
- 1 cup of coconut milk
- 1/4 tsp salt

DIRECTIONS

1. Add all ingredients into the instant pot and stir well.
2. Seal pot with lid and cook on soup mode for 30 minutes.
3. Release pressure using the quick release method than open lid carefully.
4. Puree the soup using an immersion blender until smooth.
5. Stir well and serve.

NUTRITION VALUES: Calories: 179; Total Fat: 15.6g; Saturated Fat: 13.7g; Protein: 2.8g; Carbs: 11.5g; Fiber: 4.4g; Sugar: 6.2g

68.   Broccoli Mash

Servings: 4

Preparation time: 10 minutes

Cooking time: 5 minutes

INGREDIENTS

- 1 lb broccoli, chopped
- 2 tbsp coconut cream
- 1/2 cup water
- 2 garlic cloves, crushed
- 1 tbsp olive oil
- 1/4 tsp pepper
- 1/4 tsp salt

DIRECTIONS

1. Add oil into the pot and set the pot on sauté mode.
2. Add garlic and sauté for 30 seconds.
3. Add remaining ingredients except coconut cream and stir well.
4. Seal pot with lid and cook on high for 1 minute.
5. Release pressure using quick release method than open the lid.
6. Mash the broccoli mixture using masher until smooth.
7. Stir in coconut cream. Season with pepper and salt.
8. Serve and enjoy.

NUTRITION VALUES: Calories: 88; Total Fat: 5.7g; Saturated Fat: 2.1g; Protein: 3.5g; Carbs: 8.5g; Fiber: 3.2g; Sugar: 2.2g

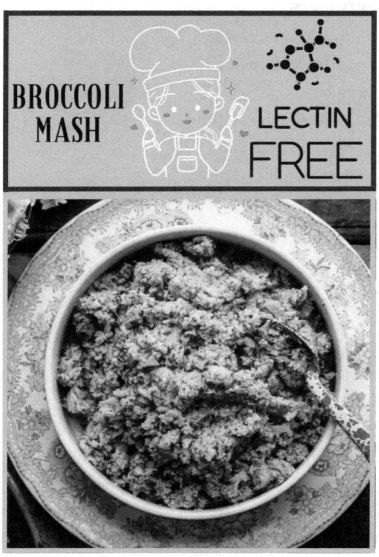

69.   Creamy Cauliflower Soup

Servings: 6

Preparation time: 10 minutes

Cooking time: 10 minutes

INGREDIENTS

- 1 lb cauliflower florets
- 3 garlic cloves, minced
- 1 onion, sliced
- 3 cups vegetable stock
- 1 cup of coconut milk
- 1 tbsp olive oil
- 2 tsp salt

DIRECTIONS

1. Add oil into the instant pot and set the pot on sauté mode.
2. Add onion into the pot and sauté until softened.
3. Add cauliflower and garlic and sauté for 5 minutes.
4. Pour coconut milk and stock into the instant pot and stir well.
5. Seal pot with lid and cook on soup mode for 5 minutes.
6. Allow to release pressure naturally then open the lid.
7. Puree the soup using an immersion blender until smooth.
8. Serve and enjoy.

NUTRITION VALUES: Calories: 142; Total Fat: 12.3g; Saturated Fat: 9.1g; Protein: 2.7g; Carbs: 8.8g; Fiber: 3.2g; Sugar: 4.3g

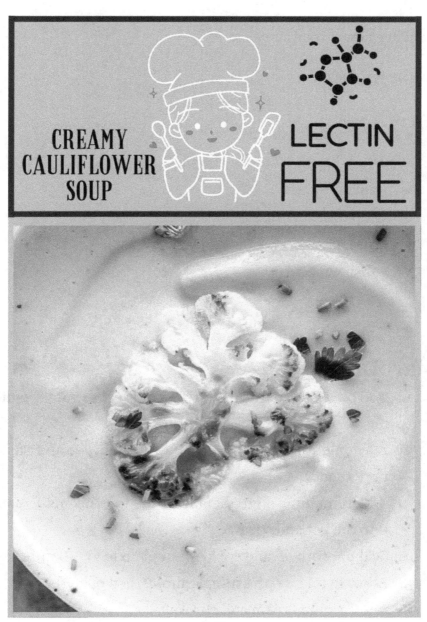

70.   Healthy Carrot Broccoli Soup

Servings: 4

Preparation time: 10 minutes

Cooking time: 30 minutes

INGREDIENTS

- 2 small carrots, diced
- 2 celery stalk, sliced
- 2 cups broccoli florets, chopped
- 1 onion, diced
- 1 cup coconut cream
- 32 oz vegetable broth
- 2 tbsp olive oil
- 1/2 tsp pepper
- 1/2 tsp salt

DIRECTIONS

1. Add olive oil into the instant pot and set the pot on sauté mode.
2. Add onion, carrots, and celery into the pot and sauté until tender.
3. Add remaining ingredients except for coconut cream into the pot and stir well.
4. Seal pot with lid and cook on soup mode for 30 minutes.
5. Allow to release pressure naturally then open the lid.
6. Add coconut cream and stir well.

7. Serve and enjoy.

NUTRITION VALUES: Calories: 273; Total Fat: 22.8g; Saturated Fat: 14g; Protein: 7.8g; Carbs: 12.7g; Fiber: 3.9g; Sugar: 5.9g

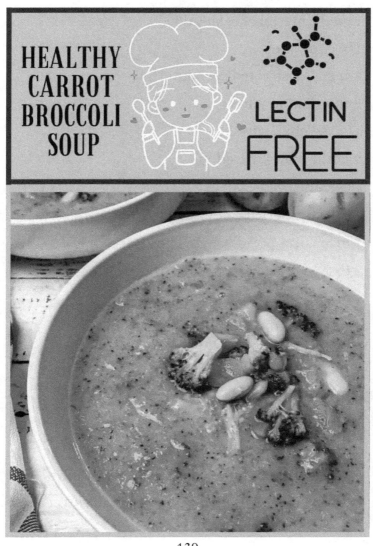

71. Lemon Coconut Cabbage

Servings: 4

Preparation time: 10 minutes

Cooking time: 19 minutes

INGREDIENTS

- 1 medium cabbage, shredded
- 1/3 cup water
- 1/2 cup desiccated coconut
- 2 tbsp lemon juice
- 1/2 red chili, sliced
- 2 garlic cloves, diced
- 1 carrot, sliced
- 1 tbsp turmeric powder
- 1 tbsp curry powder
- 1 tbsp mustard seeds
- 1 onion, sliced
- 1 tbsp olive oil
- 1 1/2 tsp salt

DIRECTIONS

1. Add oil into the instant pot and set the pot on sauté mode.
2. Add onion and salt and sauté for 2-3 minutes.
3. Add spices, chili, and garlic and stir for 30 seconds.

4. Add carrots, cabbage, coconut, and lime juice. Stir well.

5. Pour water into the pot and stir well.

6. Seal pot with lid and cook on high for 5 minutes.

7. Allow to release pressure naturally for 10 minutes then release using the quick release method.

8. Stir and serve.

NUTRITION VALUES: Calories: 162; Total Fat: 8.5g; Saturated Fat: 1.3g; Protein: 4.5g; Carbs: 20.9g; Fiber: 8g; Sugar: 9.6g

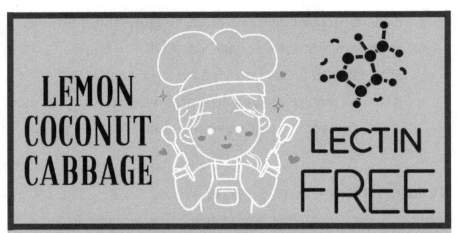

LEMON COCONUT CABBAGE

LECTIN FREE

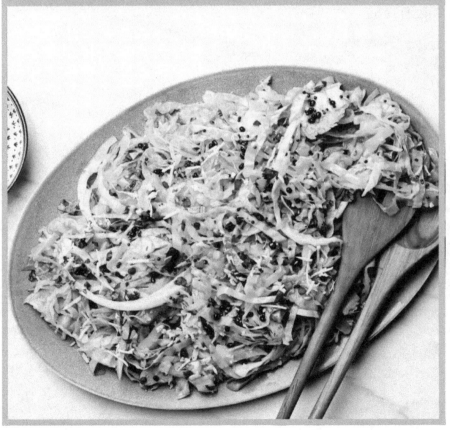

72. **Easy Cauliflower Rice**

Servings: 4

Preparation time: 10 minutes

Cooking time: 3 minutes

INGREDIENTS

- 1 medium cauliflower head, cut into florets
- 2 tbsp olive oil
- 1/4 tsp chili powder
- 1/4 tsp turmeric
- 1/4 tsp cumin
- 1/2 tsp dried parsley
- 1/4 tsp salt

DIRECTIONS

1. Pour 1 cup of water into the instant pot then place steamer basket in the pot.
2. Add cauliflower florets into the steamer basket.
3. Seal pot with lid and cook on manual high pressure for 1 minute.
4. Release pressure using quick release method than open the lid.
5. Remove cauliflower from pot and place on a dish.
6. Remove water from the instant pot.
7. Add olive oil into the pot and set the pot on sauté mode.

8. Add cooked cauliflower florets to the instant pot and stir well.

9. Break the cauliflower using potato masher into the small pieces.

10. Add remaining ingredients and stir well and cook on sauté mode for 1-2 minutes.

11. Serve and enjoy.

NUTRITION VALUES: Calories: 97; Total Fat: 7.2g; Saturated Fat: 1g; Protein: 2.9g; Carbs: 7.9g; Fiber: 3.7g; Sugar: 3.5g

73. **Simple Braised Cabbage**

Servings: 2

Preparation time: 10 minutes

Cooking time: 8 minutes

INGREDIENTS

- 1 1/2 lbs cabbage, sliced into strips
- 1 tbsp olive oil
- 1 onion, sliced
- 1/2 cup vegetable stock

DIRECTIONS

1. Add oil into the pot and set the pot on sauté mode.
2. Add onion and sauté for 5 minutes.
3. Add cabbage and stock and stir well.
4. Seal pot with lid and cook on high for 3 minutes.
5. Release pressure using quick release method than open the lid.
6. Stir well and serve.

NUTRITION VALUES: Calories: 170; Total Fat: 7.9g; Saturated Fat: 1.6g; Protein: 5g; Carbs: 25.4g; Fiber: 9.7g; Sugar: 13.7g

74.   **Mint Baby Carrots**

Servings: 4

Preparation time: 5 minutes

Cooking time: 3 minutes

INGREDIENTS

- 16 oz baby carrots
- 1 tbsp olive oil
- 1 tbsp fresh mint leaves, chopped
- 1 cup of water
- Sea salt

DIRECTIONS

1. Add carrots and water into the instant pot.
2. Seal pot with lid and cook on high for 2 minutes.
3. Release pressure using quick release method than open the lid.
4. Drain carrots well. Clean the instant pot.
5. Add olive oil and mint into the pot and sauté for 30 seconds.
6. Return carrots to the pot and season with salt.
7. Stir well and serve.

NUTRITION VALUES: Calories: 70; Total Fat: 3.7g; Saturated Fat: 0.5g; Protein: 0.8g; Carbs: 9.5g; Fiber: 3.4g; Sugar: 5.4g

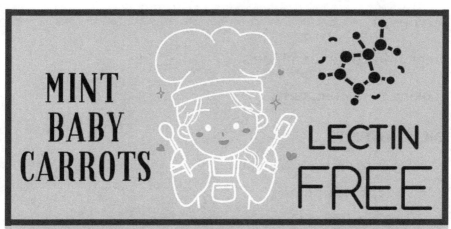

MINT BABY CARROTS

LECTIN FREE

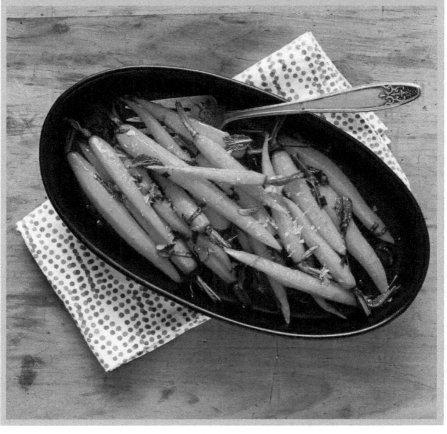

75. **Healthy Spinach Soup**

Servings: 2

Preparation time: 10 minutes

Cooking time: 10 minutes

INGREDIENTS

- 3 cups spinach, chopped
- 1 tsp garlic powder
- 2 tbsp olive oil
- ½ cup coconut cream
- 3 cups chicken broth
- 1 cup cauliflower, chopped
- ½ tsp black pepper
- ¼ tsp sea salt

DIRECTIONS

1. Add olive oil into the instant pot and set the pot on sauté mode.
2. Add cauliflower, spinach, garlic powder, pepper, and salt to the pot and stir well.
3. Add broth and stir well.
4. Seal pot with lid and cook on manual high pressure for 10 minutes.
5. Allow to release pressure naturally for 10 minutes then release using the quick release method.

6. Puree the soup using an immersion blender until smooth.

7. Stir in coconut cream. Season with pepper and salt.

8. Serve and enjoy.

NUTRITION VALUES: Calories: 344; Total Fat: 30.6g; Saturated Fat: 15.3g; Protein: 11.2g; Carbs: 10.3g; Fiber: 3.8g; Sugar: 4.8g

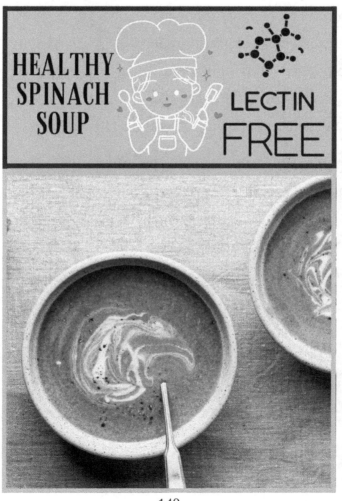

76.   Peppers and Lentils Salad

Preparation time: **10 minutes**

Cooking time: **0 minutes**

Servings: **4**

INGREDIENTS

- 14 ounces canned lentils, drained and rinsed
- 2 spring onions, chopped
- 1 red bell pepper, chopped
- 1 green bell pepper, chopped
- 1 tablespoon fresh lime juice
- 1/3 cup coriander, chopped
- 2 teaspoon balsamic vinegar

DIRECTIONS

1. In a salad bowl, combine the lentils with the onions, bell peppers and the rest of the ingredients, toss and serve.

NUTRITION VALUES: Calories 200, Fat 2.45, Fiber 6.7, Carbs 10.5, Protein 5.6

Peppers and Lentils Salad

LECTIN FREE

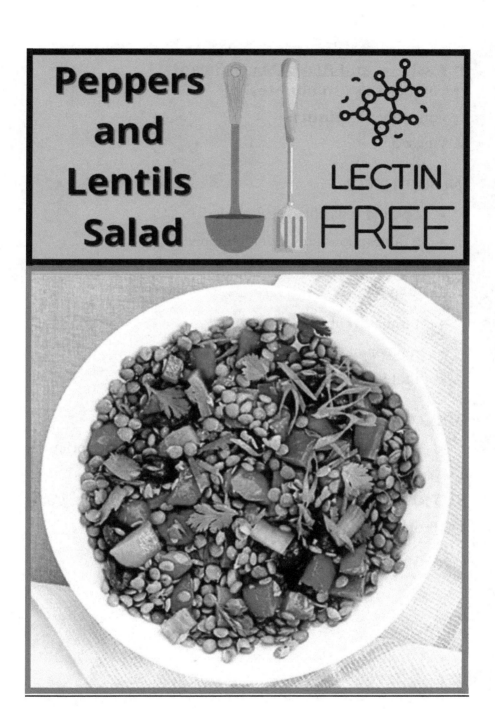

77. Cashews and Red Cabbage Salad

Preparation time: **10 minutes**

Cooking time: **0 minutes**

Servings: **4**

INGREDIENTS

- 1 pound red cabbage, shredded
- 2 tablespoons coriander, chopped
- ½ cup cashews, halved
- 2 tablespoons olive oil
- 1 tomato, cubed
- A pinch of salt and black pepper
- 1 tablespoon white vinegar

DIRECTIONS

1. In a salad bowl, combine the cabbage with the coriander and the rest of the ingredients, toss and serve cold.

NUTRITION VALUES: Calories 210, Fat 6.3, Fiber 5.2, Carbs 5.5, Protein 8

78. Apples and Pomegranate Salad

Preparation time: **10 minutes**

Cooking time: **0 minutes**

Servings: **4**

INGREDIENTS

- 3 big apples, cored and cubed
- 1 cup pomegranate seeds
- 3 cups baby arugula
- 1 cup walnuts, chopped
- 1 tablespoon olive oil
- 1 teaspoon white sesame seeds
- 2 tablespoons apple cider vinegar
- Salt and black pepper to the taste

DIRECTIONS

1. In a bowl, mix the apples with the arugula and the rest of the ingredients, toss and serve cold.

NUTRITION VALUES: Calories 160, Fat 4.3, Fiber 5.3, Carbs 8.7, Protein 10

79.   Cranberry Bulgur Mix

Preparation time: **10 minutes**

Cooking time: **0 minutes**

Servings: **4**

INGREDIENTS

- 1 and ½ cups hot water
- 1 cup bulgur
- Juice of ½ lemon
- 4 tablespoons cilantro, chopped
- ½ cup cranberries, chopped
- 1 and ½ teaspoons curry powder
- ¼ cup green onions, chopped
- ½ cup red bell peppers, chopped
- ½ cup carrots, grated
- 1 tablespoon olive oil
- A pinch of salt and black pepper

DIRECTIONS

1. Put bulgur into a bowl, add the water, stir, cover, leave aside for 10 minutes, fluff with a fork and transfer to a bowl.
2. Add the rest of the ingredients, toss, and serve cold.

NUTRITION VALUES: Calories 300, Fat 6.4, Fiber 6.1, Carbs 7.6, Protein 13

Cranberry Bulgur Mix

LECTIN FREE

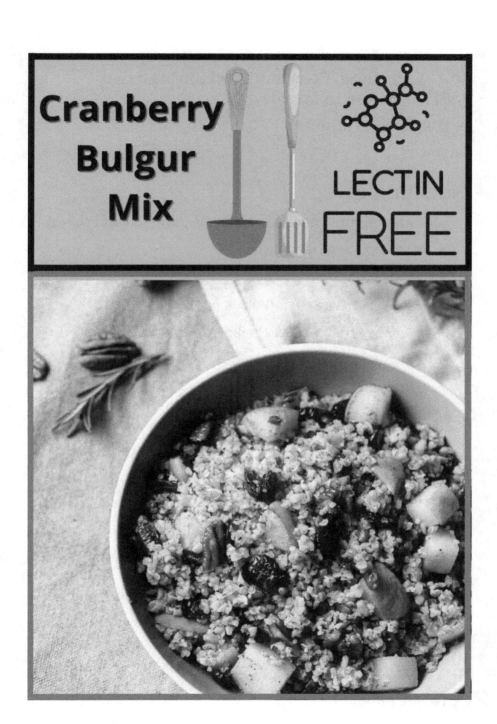

80. Chickpeas, Corn and Black Beans Salad

Preparation time: **10 minutes**

Cooking time: **0 minutes**

Servings: **4**

INGREDIENTS

- 1 and ½ cups canned black beans, drained and rinsed
- ½ teaspoon garlic powder
- 2 teaspoons chili powder
- A pinch of sea salt and black pepper
- 1 and ½ cups canned chickpeas, drained and rinsed
- 1 cup baby spinach
- 1 avocado, pitted, peeled and chopped
- 1 cup corn kernels, chopped
- 2 tablespoons lemon juice
- 1 tablespoon olive oil
- 1 tablespoon apple cider vinegar
- 1 teaspoon chives, chopped

DIRECTIONS

1. In a salad bowl, combine the black beans with the garlic powder, chili powder and the rest of the ingredients, toss and serve cold.

NUTRITION VALUES: Calories 300, Fat 13.4, Fiber 4.1, Carbs 8.6, Protein 13

81. Olives and Lentils Salad

Preparation time: **10 minutes**

Cooking time: **0 minutes**

Servings: **2**

INGREDIENTS

- 1/3 cup canned green lentils, drained and rinsed
- 1 tablespoon olive oil
- 2 cups baby spinach
- 1 cup black olives, pitted and halved
- 2 tablespoons sunflower seeds
- 1 tablespoon Dijon mustard
- 2 tablespoons balsamic vinegar
- 2 tablespoons olive oil

DIRECTIONS

1. In a bowl, mix the lentils with the spinach, olives and the rest of the ingredients, toss and serve cold.

NUTRITION VALUES: Calories 279, Fat 6.5, Fiber 4.5, Carbs 9.6, Protein 12

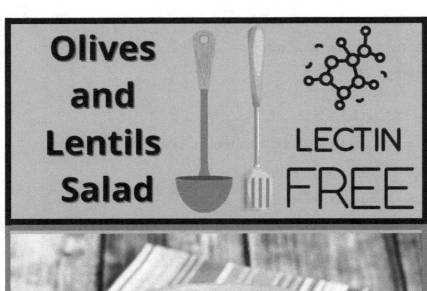

Olives and Lentils Salad

LECTIN FREE

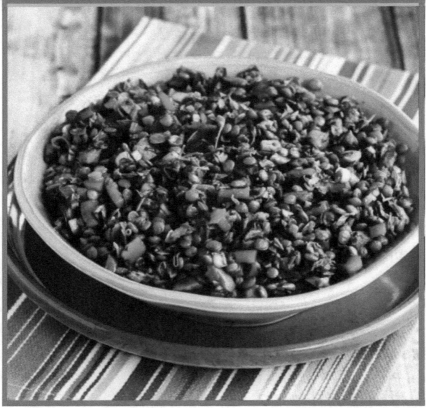

82. **Coconut Celery Soup**

Servings: 4

Preparation time: 10 minutes

Cooking time: 30 minutes

INGREDIENTS

- 6 cups celery stalk, chopped
- 2 cups vegetable stock
- 1 onion, chopped
- 1/2 tsp dill
- 1 cup of coconut milk
- 1/4 tsp salt

DIRECTIONS

6. Add all ingredients into the instant pot and stir well.
7. Seal pot with lid and cook on soup mode for 30 minutes.
8. Release pressure using the quick release method than open lid carefully.
9. Puree the soup using an immersion blender until smooth.
10. Stir well and serve.

NUTRITION VALUES: Calories: 179; Total Fat: 15.6g; Saturated Fat: 13.7g; Protein: 2.8g; Carbs: 11.5g; Fiber: 4.4g; Sugar: 6.2g

SNACKS

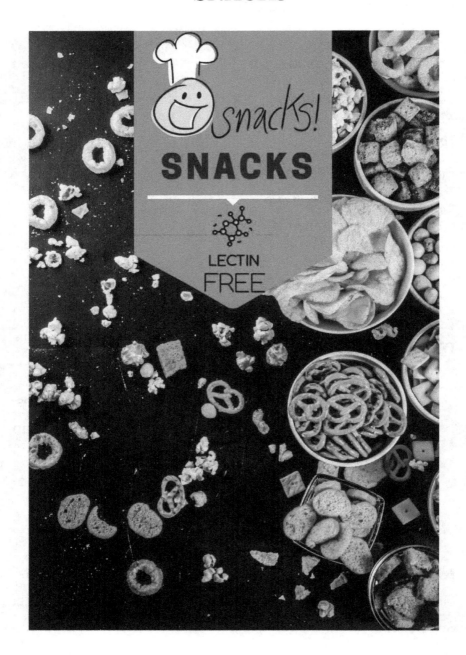

83. **Coated Chicken Wings**

Preparation Time: 10 minutes

Cooking time: 8 minutes

Servings: 4

INGREDIENTS

- 4 chicken wings, skinless
- 2 oz pork rind, chopped
- 1 egg, whisked
- 1 teaspoon olive oil
- 1 teaspoon paprika
- ¾ teaspoon chili flakes
- ½ teaspoon turmeric
- 1 teaspoon butter
- ½ teaspoon salt

DIRECTIONS

1. Sprinkle the chicken wings with chili flakes, turmeric, paprika, and salt.
2. Then dip them in the whisked egg and coat in the almond flour.
3. Pour olive oil in the pan and preheat it.
4. Place the coated chicken wings in the pan and cook them for 4 minutes from each side over the medium heat.
5. Then transfer the chicken wings on the plate. It is recommended to eat chicken wings hot.

NUTRITION VALUES: calories 395, fat 19.2, fiber 0.3, carbs 0.6, protein 52.9

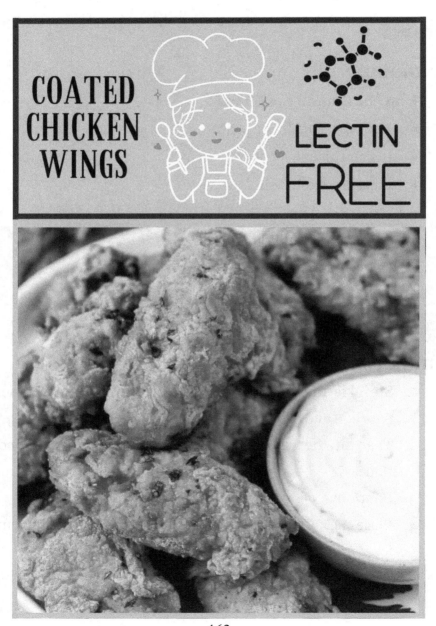

84. **Cheese Plate with Marinated Peppers**

Preparation Time: 15 minutes

Servings: 6

INGREDIENTS

- 3 oz Provolone cheese, chopped
- 2 oz Cheddar cheese, chopped
- 3 oz Swiss cheese, chopped
- 3 oz Parmesan cheese, chopped
- 1 bell pepper
- 1 jalapeno pepper, minced
- 1 tablespoon olive oil
- 1 teaspoon apple cider vinegar
- ½ teaspoon ground black pepper
- ½ teaspoon ground coriander
- 3 tablespoons water

DIRECTIONS

1. Put the cheese on the serving plate by rows.
2. In the separated bowl, whisk together minced jalapeno pepper, olive oil, apple cider vinegar, ground black pepper, and ground coriander.
3. Remove the seeds from bell pepper and chop it.
4. Add it in the minced jalapeno mixture.
5. Add 3 tablespoons of water. Whisk it.

6. Sprinkle the mixture over the cheese cubes. Pin the cheese with toothpicks for comfortable eating.

NUTRITION VALUES: calories 215, fat 16.3, fiber 0.4, carbs 3.5, protein 14.6

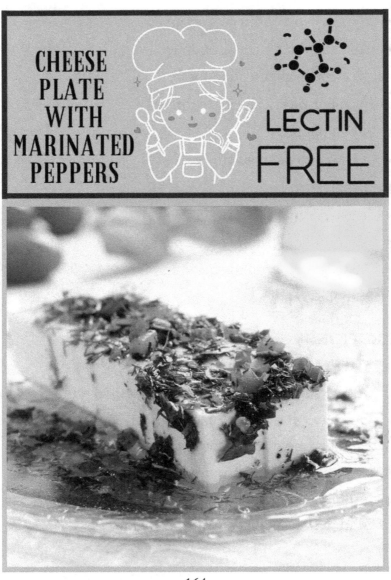

85.   Lectin Free Chocolate Mousse

Cooking Time: 50 Min

Preparation Time: 5 Minutes

Servings:2

INGREDIENTS

- 2 cans full-fat coconut milk, refrigerated for 24 hours
- 2 tablespoons raw cocoa powder, organic
- 4 tablespoons granular sweetener, unsweetened

HOW TO

- Take out the coconut can from the refrigerator and scoop out it's hardened part and place it in a mixing bowl; use the water part of the coconut milk for further use.
- Next, add in the sweetener and cocoa powder in the bowl and whisk it on a high speed until it gets peaks and a consistency of mousse.
- Finally, transfer it in a bowl serve chilled with sprinkles of grated coconut.

NUTRITION   VALUE: Calories: 138   Fat: 11.7g
Carbohydrates: 20g Protein: 2g

86.   Vegan Superfood Ice Cream

Cooking Time: 10 Min

Preparation Time: 5 Minutes

Servings:4

INGREDIENTS

- 2 cans full fat coconut milk, organic and refrigerated for 24 hours
- 4 teaspoons moringa powder
- 1 tablespoon granular sweetener, unsweetened
- 2 teaspoons baobab powder, organic
- 1 cup cocoa nibs, organic

HOW TO

- Pour all the ingredients in a blender and mix till it gets very fine and smooth consistency.
- Ad d in the sweetener as told or as per your choice.
- Next, pour in the ice cream mixture in an ice cream maker and make ice cream as per the machine's directions.
- Mix in the cocoa nibs and refrigerate it for 1 hour.
- Take it out from the refrigerator and scoop it out in a bowl.
- Enjoy eating!

NUTRITION   VALUE: Calories: 293   Fat: 27.4g
Carbohydrates: 16.7g Protein: 4g

87. **Chocolate Covered Strawberry Truffles**

Cooking Time: 40 Min

Preparation Time: 30 Minutes

Servings:12

INGREDIENTS

For Truffles:

- 4 cups strawberries, dried and organic
- 16 medjool dates, large and pitted

For Coating:

- 2 teaspoons coconut oil, organic
- ½ cup enjoy Life 69% Cocoa Dark Chocolate Morsels

HOW TO:

- Take a food processor and put all the ingredients of truffle in it; pulse until it gets a crumbly and muggy texture.
- Now, scoop some mixture into your hands and form gold size balls out of it.
- Next, for chocolate coating take a pan over the stove and put coconut oil and cocoa chocolate morsels into it; mix till it forms a smooth consistency.
- Finally dip the strawberry truffles into the chocolate mixture and place them all in the refrigerator for about 20 minutes or till the chocolate hardens.
- Upon chilling, enjoy!

NUTRITION VALUE: Calories: 154 Fat: 3.4g Carbohydrates: 32.6g Protein: 1.5g

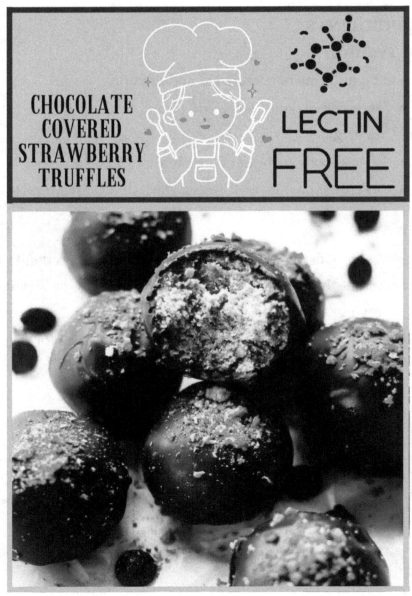

88. **Cauliflower Rice Pudding**

Cooking Time: 30 Min

Preparation Time: 10 Minutes

Servings:4

INGREDIENTS

- 1 pound cauliflower head, small, processed in food processor
- 3 cups coconut milk
- 1 cup coconut flakes, unsweetened, powdered
- 1 tablespoon vanilla extract, pure
- ½ teaspoon sea salt
- 1 teaspoon raw honey
- Pinch nutmeg

HOW TO:

- In a heavy bottom skillet put some coconut oil.
- Add in the cauliflower rice and give it a mix for 15 minutes.
- Transfer it to a plate for further use.
- Now in the same skillet add in some coconut milk along with vanilla, powdered coconut flakes, honey, salt and nutmeg; give it a good mix and allow it to cook for 15 minutes.
- Finally add in the fried cauliflower rice into the coconut milk mixture and allow it to cook for 5 minutes, until thickened.

- Serve it in a bowl and enjoy eating!

NUTRITION VALUE: Calories: 528 Total Fat: 49.7g Carbohydrates: 20.9g Protein: 7g

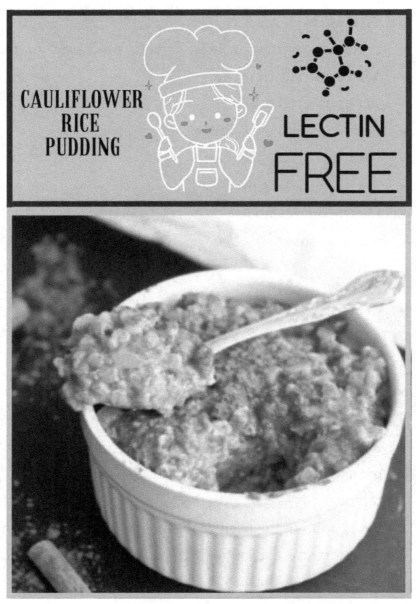

89. __Chocolate Mint Brownies__

Cooking Time: 25 Min

Preparation Time: 15 Minutes

Servings:4

INGREDIENTS

- ¼ cup macadamia nuts
- ¼ cup fresh mint
- ¼ teaspoon baking soda
- ½ cup coconut oil
- 3 ounces bittersweet chocolate, chunks
- 2 tablespoons erythritol
- 1 ½ tablespoon coconut flour
- 1 tablespoon peppermint extract
- 3 large pastured eggs

HOW TO

1. Take a food processor and add in the macadamia nuts, mint and baking soda in it; process.
2. Next, add in the coconut oil along with bittersweet chocolate, erythritol, coconut flour, omega eggs and peppermint extract; process again.
3. Grease a heat proof flat dish and pour the batter in it.
4. Take an electric pressure cooker and place a trivet in it; place the heat proof dish on the trivet and pressure cook the brownie bar after closing the lid of the cooker for 30 minutes almost.

5. After the timer goes off, quick release the pressure naturally and open the lid.

6. Next, release the bar from the mould and cut it into smaller chunks.

7. Serve it on the plate and enjoy eating.

NUTRITION VALUE: Calories: 473 Total Fat: 43.3 g Carbohydrates: 23 g Protein: 7 g

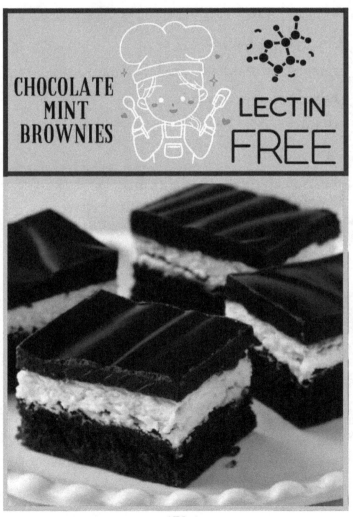

90.   **Sausage Skewers**
Preparation Time: 15 minutes

Cooking time: 6 minutes

Servings:4

INGREDIENTS

- 1 cup ground beef
- 1 zucchini, roughly chopped
- 1 teaspoon ground black pepper
- 1 teaspoon apple cider vinegar
- ½ teaspoon salt
- 1 teaspoon turmeric

DIRECTIONS

1. In mixing bowl, mix up together ground beef, ground black pepper, and salt.
2. Make the small balls (sausages).
3. Then string beef balls and chopped zucchini one-by-one in the skewers.
4. Sprinkle the skewers with apple cider vinegar and turmeric.
5. Preheat the grill to 365F.
6. Place the skewers in the grill and cook them for 6 minutes. Flip them into another side from time to time.
7. Always serve the skewers only hot.

NUTRITION VALUES: calories 76, fat 4.3, fiber 0.8, carbs 2.4, protein 7.2

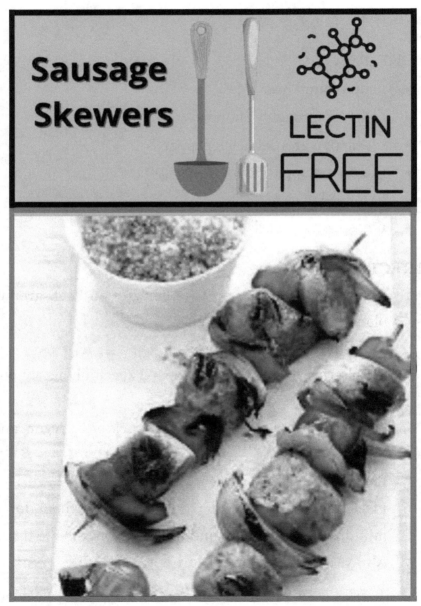

91. Keto Crackers

Preparation Time: 15 minutes

Cooking time: 15 minutes

Servings: 9

INGREDIENTS

- 1 cup coconut flour
- ½ cup almond flour
- 1 tablespoon flax seeds
- ¾ teaspoon salt
- 1 teaspoon smoked paprika
- 1 teaspoon sesame seeds
- 1 tablespoon olive oil
- ¼ cup of water

DIRECTIONS

1. In the mixing bowl, combine together coconut flour, almond flour, flax seeds, salt, smoked paprika, and olive oil. Add water.
2. Knead the soft and non-sticky dough.
3. Roll up the dough and sprinkle it with sesame seeds.
4. Press the seeds in the dough.
5. Cut the dough into crackers.
6. Line the baking tray with parchment. Place the crackers on the parchment.
7. Preheat the oven to 355F.

8. Place the tray with crackers in the oven and cook for 15 minutes.

9. Chill the crackers well. The chilled crackers will be crunchy.

NUTRITION VALUES: calories 82, fat 4.1, fiber 5.8, carbs 9.7, protein 2.3

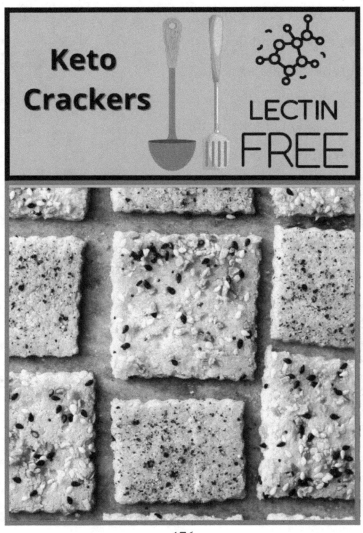

92. **Garlic Deviled Eggs**

Preparation Time: 10 minutes

Cooking time: 8 minutes

Servings: 4

INGREDIENTS

- 2 eggs
- 1 jalapeno pepper, minced
- ½ teaspoon cream cheese
- ½ teaspoon minced garlic
- ¼ teaspoon white pepper
- ¾ teaspoon salt
- 1 teaspoon butter
- 1 cup water, for cooking

DIRECTIONS

1. Pour water in the saucepan, add eggs.
2. Boil the eggs for 8 minutes.
3. Meanwhile, combine together cream cheese, minced garlic, white pepper, salt, and butter. Churn the mixture until soft and smooth.
4. When the eggs are cooked, chill them in ice water and peel.
5. Cut the eggs into the halves.
6. Add the cooked egg yolks in the cream cheese mixture. Mix it up.

7. Fill the egg whites with the garlic mass.

NUTRITION VALUES: calories 43, fat 3.3, fiber 0.1, carbs 0.6, protein 2.9

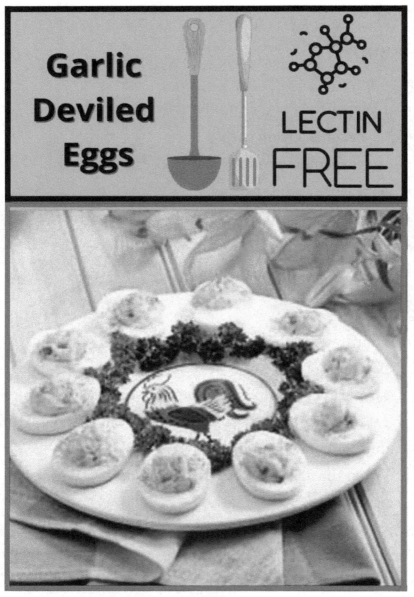

93.   **Fried Mushroom Bombs**

Preparation Time: 15 minutes

Cooking time: 25 minutes

Servings: 8

INGREDIENTS

- ½ cup mushrooms
- 1 white onion, diced
- 1 cup ground pork
- 2 tablespoons almond flour
- 1 teaspoon salt
- 1 tablespoon butter
- 1 egg, beaten
- 1 tablespoon coconut flour
- 1 teaspoon dried oregano
- 4 tablespoons water

DIRECTIONS

1. Finely chop the mushrooms and put them in the skillet.
2. Add diced onion, butter, salt, and dried oregano.
3. Cook the vegetables for 10 minutes over the medium heat.
4. Meanwhile, mix up together ground pork, almond flour, and beaten egg. Mix up the mixture well.

5. Add the cooked vegetables in the ground pork mixture. Mix it up again.

6. Make the medium size balls from the meat mass and sprinkle them with coconut flour.

7. Place the bombs in the tray, add water and transfer in the preheated to the 365F oven.

8. Cook the mushroom bombs for 15 minutes. Stir them gently after 7 minutes of cooking.

NUTRITION VALUES: calories 135, fat 10.1, fiber 1.5, carbs 3.6, protein 8.1

94.   **<u>Spinach Dip</u>**

Preparation Time: 7 minutes

Cooking time: 15 minutes

Servings: 8

INGREDIENTS

- 1 ½ cup spinach, chopped
- 4 oz artichoke hearts, canned
- 3 tablespoons cream cheese
- 1 tablespoon butter
- 3 oz Swiss cheese, grated
- ¼ cup coconut cream
- 1 teaspoon garlic powder
- ½ teaspoon chili flakes

DIRECTIONS

1. Place spinach in the saucepan.
2. Add cream cheese, butter, garlic powder, and chili flakes.
3. Saute the greens for 5 minutes over the medium heat.
4. Meanwhile, chop the artichoke hearts.
5. Add then in the spinach and mix up well.
6. Add coconut cream and stir well. Saute the sip for 5 minutes more
7. After this, add grated Swiss cheese and mix up the dip well.

8. When the spinach dip is homogenous and smooth, it is cooked.

9. It is recommended to serve the meal warm or hot.

NUTRITION VALUES: calories 93, fat 7.5, fiber 1.1, carbs 3, protein 4

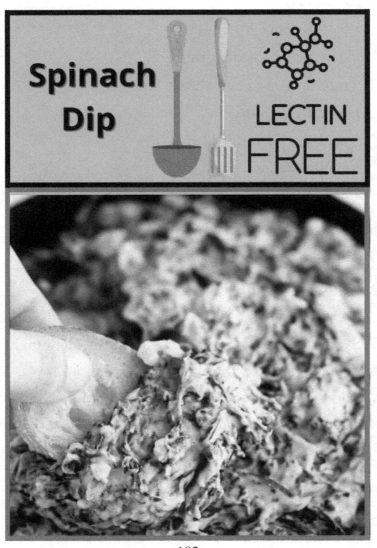

95. **Spicy Crab Dip**

Preparation Time: 15 minutes

Cooking time: 20 minutes

Servings: 8

INGREDIENTS

- 7 oz crab meat, canned
- 1 white onion, minced
- 1 teaspoon onion powder
- 2 tablespoons mayonnaise
- ¼ cup heavy cream
- 5 oz Cheddar cheese
- ½ teaspoon salt
- 1 teaspoon ground paprika
- 1 teaspoon dried thyme

DIRECTIONS

1. Chop the crab meat and put it in the casserole dish.
2. Add minced white onion, onion powder, salt, ground paprika, and dried thyme. Mix it up.
3. Shred the cheese.
4. Add mayonnaise and heavy cream in the crabmeat mixture. Stir it gently.
5. Then sprinkle the crab meat mixture with the shredded cheese and cover with foil. Secure the edges of the casserole dish.

6. Cook the dip in the preheated to 365F oven for 20 minutes.

NUTRITION VALUES: calories 129, fat 9, fiber 0.5, carbs 3.4, protein 7.9

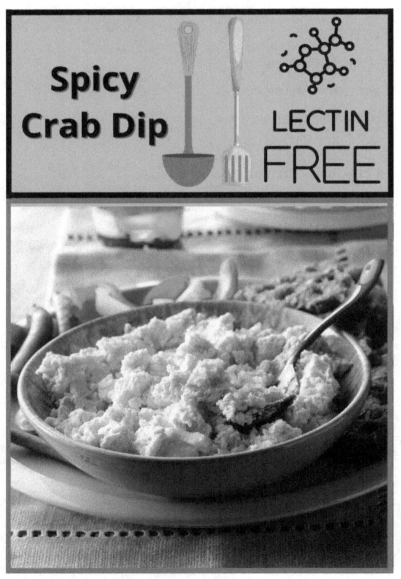

DESSERTS

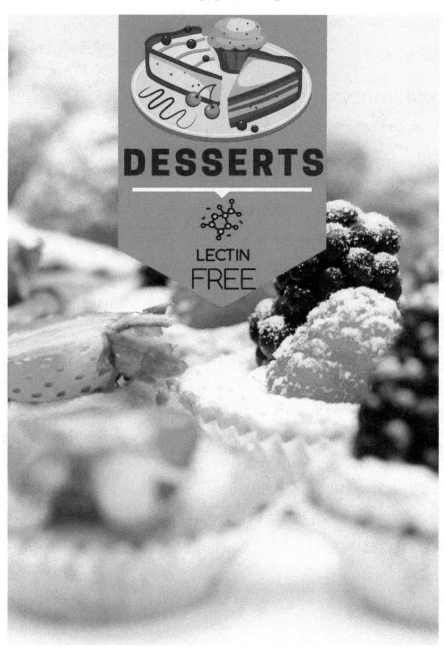

96. Vanilla Keto Ice Cream

Preparation Time: 3 hours 10 minutes

Servings: 6

INGREDIENTS

- 4 eggs; yolks and whites separated
- 1/2 cup swerve
- 1¼ cup heavy whipping cream
- 1 tablespoon vanilla extract
- 1/4 teaspoon cream of tartar

DIRECTIONS

1. In a bowl, mix egg whites with cream of tartar and swerve and stir using your mixer.
2. In another bowl, whisk cream with vanilla extract and blend very well.
3. Combine the 2 mixtures and stir gently.
4. In another bowl, whisk egg yolks very well and then add the two egg whites mix.
5. Stir gently, pour this into a container and keep in the freezer for 3 hours before serving your ice cream.

NUTRITION VALUES: Calories: 243; Fat 22; Fiber 0; Carbs 2; Protein 4

97. __Jello Dessert__

Preparation Time: 2 hours 15 minutes

Servings: 12

INGREDIENTS

- 2 ounces packets sugar free jello
- 1 teaspoon vanilla extract
- 3 tablespoons erythritol
- 1 cup cold water
- 1 cup hot water
- 1 cup heavy cream
- 1 cup boiling water
- 2 tablespoons gelatin powder

DIRECTIONS

1. Put jello packets in a bowl, add 1 cup hot water; stir until it dissolves and then mix with 1 cup cold water.
2. Pour this into a lined square dish and keep in the fridge for 1 hour.
3. Cut into cubes and leave aside for now.
4. Meanwhile; in a bowl, mix erythritol with vanilla extract, 1 cup boiling water, gelatin and heavy cream and stir very well.
5. Pour half of this mix into a silicon round mold, spread jello cubes, then top with the rest of the gelatin.
6. Keep in the fridge for 1 more hour and then serve

NUTRITION VALUES: Calories: 70; Fat 1; Fiber 0; Carbs 1; Protein 2

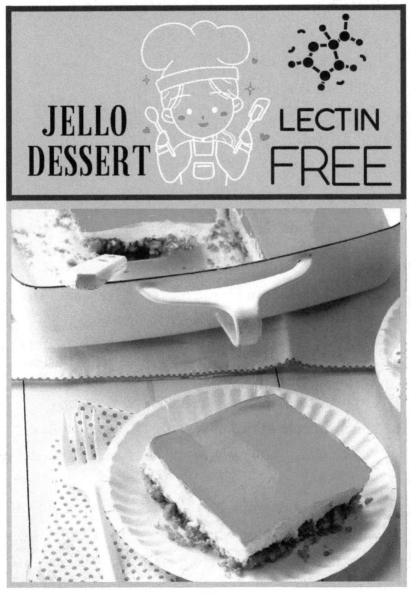

98. Keto Nutella

Preparation Time: 10 minutes

Servings: 6

INGREDIENTS

- 2 ounces coconut oil
- 4 tablespoons cocoa powder
- 1 cup walnuts; halved
- 4 tablespoons stevia
- 1 teaspoon vanilla extract

DIRECTIONS

1. In your food processor, mix cocoa powder with oil, vanilla, walnuts and stevia and blend very well.
2. Keep in the fridge for a couple of hours and then serve

NUTRITION VALUES: Calories: 100; Fat 10; Fiber 1; Carbs 3; Protein 2

99. Avocado Pudding

Preparation Time: 10 minutes

Servings: 4

INGREDIENTS

- 2 avocados; pitted, peeled and chopped.
- 1 tablespoon lime juice
- 2 teaspoons vanilla extract
- 14 ounces canned coconut milk
- 80 drops stevia

DIRECTIONS

1. In your blender, mix avocado with coconut milk, vanilla extract, stevia and lime juice, blend well, spoon into dessert bowls and keep in the fridge until you serve it.

NUTRITION VALUES: Calories: 150; Fat 3; Fiber 3; Carbs 5; Protein 6

100. **Cookie Dough Balls**

Preparation Time: 10 minutes

Servings: 10

INGREDIENTS

- 1/2 cup almond butter
- 1/2 teaspoon vanilla extract
- 3 tablespoons coconut sugar
- 1 teaspoon cinnamon; powder
- 3 tablespoons coconut flour
- 3 tablespoons coconut milk
- 15 drops vanilla stevia
- A pinch of salt

For the topping:

- 3 tablespoons granulated swerve
- 1½ teaspoon cinnamon powder

DIRECTIONS

1. In a bowl, mix almond butter with 1 teaspoon cinnamon, coconut flour, coconut milk, coconut sugar, vanilla extract, vanilla stevia and a pinch of salt and stir well.
2. Shape balls out of this mix.
3. In another bowl mix 1½ teaspoon cinnamon powder with swerve and stir well.
4. Roll balls in cinnamon mix and keep them in the fridge until you serve

NUTRITION VALUES: Calories: 89; Fat 1; Fiber 2; Carbs 4; Protein 2

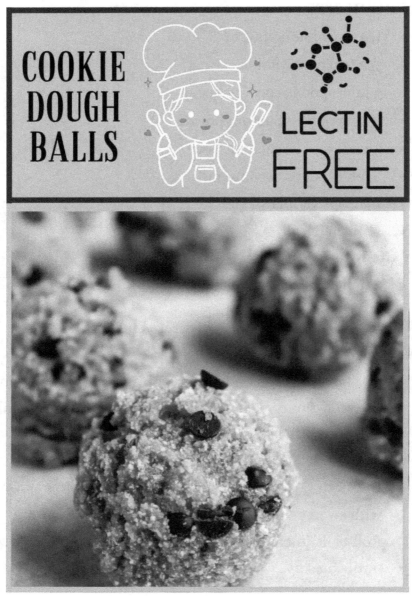

101. Chocolate Biscotti

Preparation Time: 22 minutes

Servings: 8

INGREDIENTS

- 2 cups almonds
- 1/4 cup cocoa powder
- 1/4 cup coconut oil
- 2 tablespoons chia seeds
- 1 egg
- 2 tablespoons stevia
- 1 teaspoon baking soda
- 1/4 cup coconut; shredded
- A pinch of salt

DIRECTIONS

1. In your food processor, mix chia seeds with almonds and blend well.
2. Add coconut, egg, coconut oil, cocoa powder, a pinch of salt, baking soda and stevia and blend well.
3. Shape 8 biscotti pieces out of this dough, place on a lined baking sheet, introduce in the oven at 350 degrees and bake for 12 minutes
4. Serve them warm or cold.

NUTRITION VALUES: Calories: 200; Fat 2; Fiber 1; Carbs 3; Protein 4

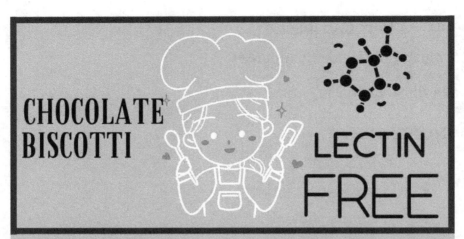

CHOCOLATE BISCOTTI

LECTIN FREE

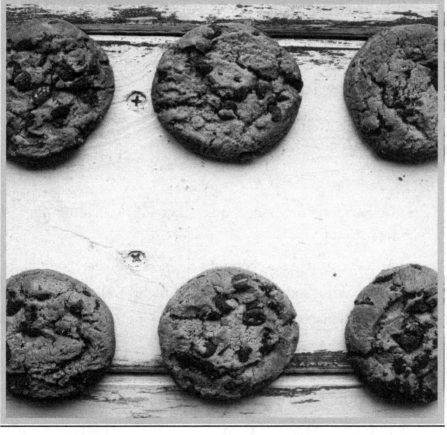

102. **Lime Cheesecake**

Preparation Time: 12 minutes

Servings: 10

INGREDIENTS

- 4 ounces almond meal
- 2 tablespoons ghee; melted
- 2 teaspoons granulated stevia
- 1/4 cup coconut; unsweetened and shredded

For the filling:

- 1 pound cream cheese
- 2 cup hot water
- 2 sachets sugar free lime jelly
- Zest from 1 lime
- Juice from 1 lime

DIRECTIONS

1. Heat up a small pan over medium heat; add ghee and stir until it melts
2. In a bowl, mix coconut with almond meal, ghee and stevia and stir well.
3. Press this on the bottom of a round pan and keep in the fridge for now.
4. Meanwhile; put hot water in a bowl, add jelly sachets and stir until it dissolves
5. Put cream cheese in a bowl, add jelly and stir very well.

6. Add lime juice and zest and blend using your mixer.

7. Pour this over base, spread and keep the cheesecake in the fridge until you serve it.

NUTRITION VALUES: Calories: 300; Fat 23; Fiber 2; Carbs 5; Protein 7

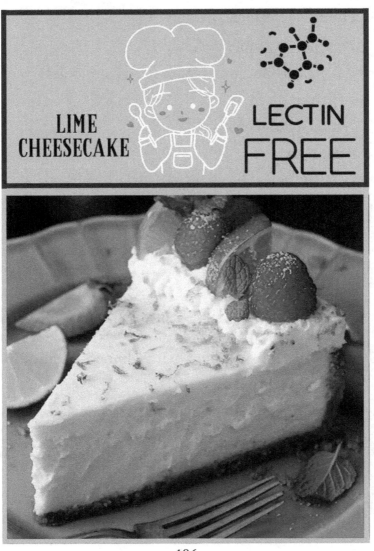

103. Keto Cherry And Chia Jam

Preparation Time: 27 minutes

Servings: 22

INGREDIENTS

- 2 ½ cups cherries; pitted
- 10 drops stevia
- 1 cup water
- 3 tablespoons chia seeds
- Peel from 1/2 lemon; grated
- 1/4 cup erythritol
- 1/2 teaspoon vanilla powder

DIRECTIONS

1. Put cherries and the water in a pot, add stevia, erythritol, vanilla powder, chia seeds and lemon peel; stir, bring to a simmer and cook for 12 minutes
2. Take off heat and then leave your jam aside for 15 minutes at least.
3. Serve cold.

NUTRITION VALUES: Calories: 60; Fat 1; Fiber 1; Carbs 2; Protein 0.5

104. **Chocolate Cookies**

Preparation Time: 50 minutes

Servings: 12

INGREDIENTS

- 1 teaspoon vanilla extract
- 1/2 cup unsweetened chocolate chips
- 1/4 cup swerve
- 1/2 cup ghee
- 1 egg
- 2 tablespoons coconut sugar
- 2 cups almond flour
- A pinch of salt

DIRECTIONS

1. Heat up a pan with the ghee over medium heat; stir and cook until it browns
2. Take this off heat and leave aside for 5 minutes
3. In a bowl, mix egg with vanilla extract, coconut sugar and swerve and stir.
4. Add melted ghee, flour, salt and half of the chocolate chips and stir everything.
5. Transfer this to a pan, spread the rest of the chocolate chips on top, introduce in the oven at 350 degrees F and bake for 30 minutes
6. Slice when it's cold and serve

NUTRITION VALUES: Calories: 230; Fat 12; Fiber 2; Carbs 4; Protein 5

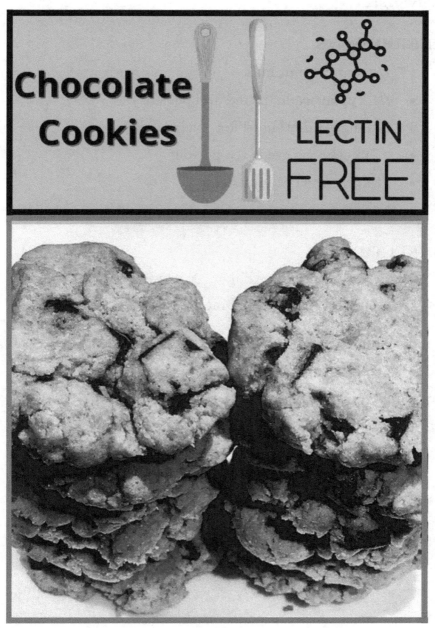

105. Dessert Smoothie
Preparation Time: 5 minutes

Servings: 2

INGREDIENTS

- 1/2 cup coconut milk
- 1½ cup avocado; pitted and peeled
- 1 mango thinly sliced for serving
- 2 tablespoons green tea powder
- 1 tablespoon coconut sugar
- 2 teaspoons lime zest

DIRECTIONS

1. In your smoothie maker, combine milk with avocado, green tea powder and lime zest and pulse well.

2. Add sugar, blend well, divide into 2 glasses and serve with mango slices on top.

NUTRITION VALUES: Calories: 87; Fat 5; Fiber 3; Carbs 6; Protein 8

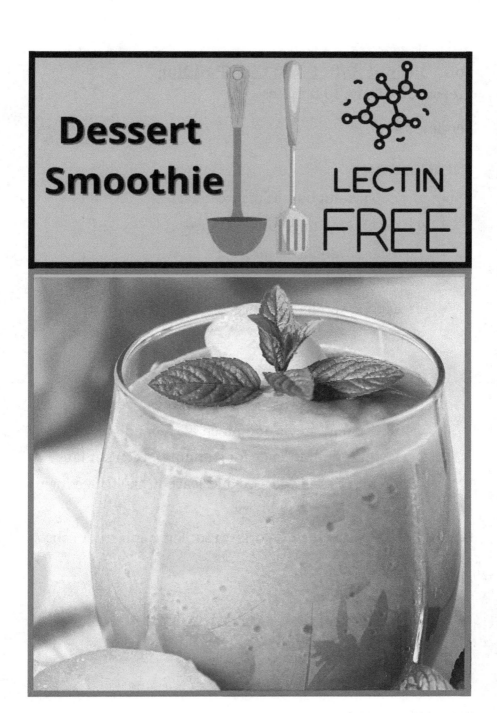

Dessert Smoothie

LECTIN FREE

106. Peanut Butter And Chia Pudding

Preparation Time: 10 minutes

Servings: 4

INGREDIENTS

- 1/4 cup peanut butter; unsweetened
- 2 cups almond milk; unsweetened
- 1 teaspoon vanilla extract
- 1/2 cup chia seeds
- 1 teaspoon vanilla stevia
- A pinch of salt

DIRECTIONS

1. In a bowl, mix milk with chia seeds, peanut butter, vanilla extract, stevia and pinch of salt and stir well.
2. Leave this pudding aside for 5 minutes, then stir it again, divide into dessert glasses and leave in the fridge for 10 minutes

NUTRITION VALUES: Calories: 120; Fat 1; Fiber 2; Carbs 4; Protein 2

107. Coconut And Strawberry Desert

Preparation Time: 10 minutes

Servings: 4

INGREDIENTS

- 1¾ cups coconut cream
- 2 teaspoons granulated stevia
- 1 cup strawberries

DIRECTIONS

1. Put coconut cream in a bowl, add stevia and stir very well using an immersion blender.
2. Add strawberries, fold them gently into the mix, divide dessert into glasses and serve them cold.

NUTRITION VALUES: Calories: 245; Fat 24; Fiber 1; Carbs 5; Protein 4

108. Ricotta Mousse

Preparation Time: 2 hours 10 minutes

Servings: 10

INGREDIENTS

- 1/2 cup hot coffee
- 2 cups ricotta cheese
- 2½ teaspoons gelatin
- 1 teaspoon espresso powder
- 1 teaspoon vanilla stevia
- 1 teaspoon vanilla extract
- 1 cup whipping cream
- A pinch of salt

DIRECTIONS

1. In a bowl, mix coffee with gelatin; stir well and leave aside until coffee is cold.
2. In a bowl, mix espresso, stevia, salt, vanilla extract and ricotta and stir using a mixer.
3. Add coffee mix and stir everything well.
4. Add whipping cream and blend mixture again.
5. Divide into dessert bowls and serve after you've kept it in the fridge for 2 hours

NUTRITION VALUES: Calories: 160; Fat 13; Fiber 0; Carbs 2; Protein 7

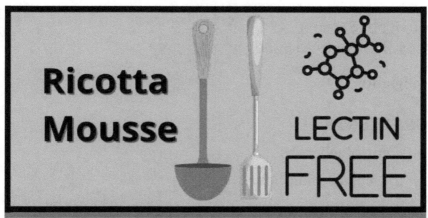

Ricotta Mousse

LECTIN FREE

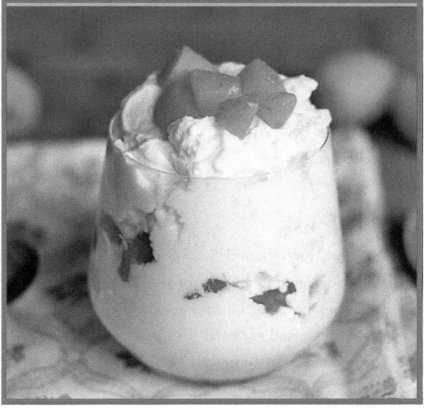

109. <u>Keto Scones</u>
Preparation Time: 20 minutes

Servings: 10

INGREDIENTS
- 1 cup blueberries
- 1/2 cup coconut flour
- 2 eggs
- 5 tablespoons stevia
- 1/2 cup ghee
- 1/2 cup almond flour
- 2 teaspoons vanilla extract
- 2 teaspoons baking powder
- 1/2 cup heavy cream
- A pinch of salt

DIRECTIONS
1. In a bowl, mix almond flour with coconut flour, salt, baking powder and blueberries and stir well.
2. In another bowl, mix heavy cream with ghee, vanilla extract, stevia and eggs and stir well.
3. Combine the 2 mixtures and stir until you obtain your dough.
4. Shape 10 triangles from this mix, place them on a lined baking sheet, introduce in the oven at 350 degrees F and bake for 10 minutes Serve them cold.

NUTRITION VALUES: Calories: 130; Fat 2; Fiber 2; Carbs 4; Protein 3

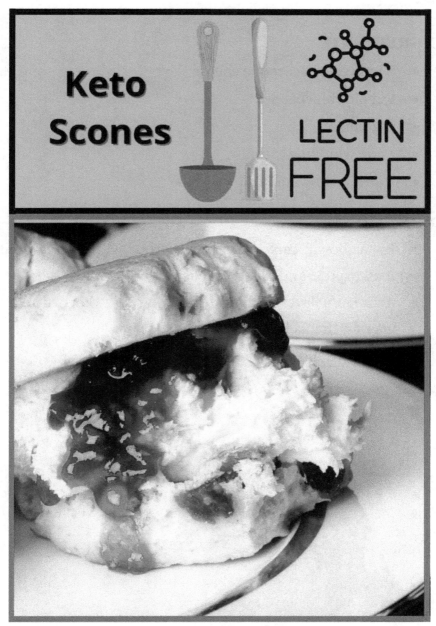

110. Delicious Mousse

Preparation Time: 10 minutes

Servings: 12

INGREDIENTS

- 8 ounces mascarpone cheese
- 1/2 pint blueberries
- 1/2 pint strawberries
- 1 cup whipping cream
- ¾ teaspoon vanilla stevia

DIRECTIONS

1. In a bowl, mix whipping cream with stevia and mascarpone and blend well using your mixer.
2. Arrange a layer of blueberries and strawberries in 12 glasses, then a layer of cream and so on.
3. Serve this mousse cold!

348mg

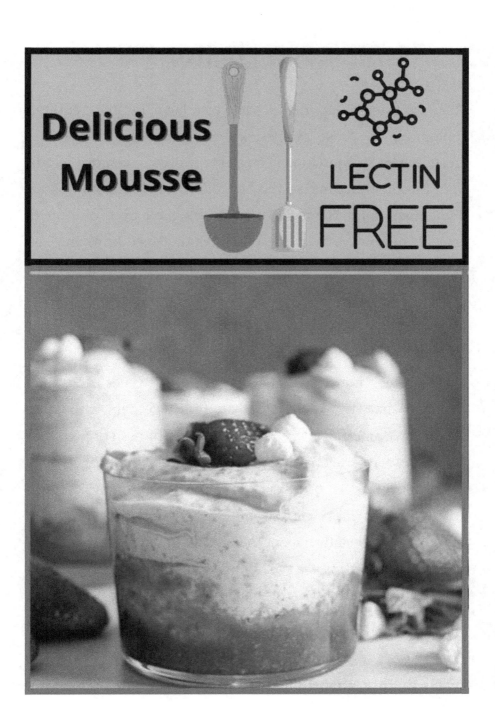

Delicious Mousse

LECTIN FREE

CONCLUSION

The next step is to make sure you have all the required appliances for these recipes, so you can begin a healthier lifestyle. Dr. Steven Gundry suggests everyone remove lectins from their diet because of the harm they can cause our bodies. Remember, may plants have been designed by evolution to protect themselves from the creatures that feed on them, i.e.: animals and insects. In humans, this causes a gastrointestinal upset like leaky gut syndrome, mild to severe abdominal pain, gas, and they may aggravate any autoimmune disorder you may have going on in your body.

Do you remember what lectins are? They are types of Protein, Overalls that tie the carbohydrates together within an organism. Sometimes this is encouraging in assisting certain particles to interact with one another at a molecular level. Sometimes this is necessary to aid in some physiological functions, but most of the time it is more harmful than anything... especially when there is a high enough level of lectins. These lectins are the hooks on any molecule that attach to other molecules. Think of this interaction almost like Velcro.

Many foods have lectins in them; just remember there are surefire ways to remove many of the lectins so that they will be unable to cause almost problems in your body. You can always soak the foods, sprout them, soak them, ferment them, or pressure-cook them. The possibilities are endless with a little bit of effort. It is a shame for anyone to have to experience a life without comfort. You could have a life with no stomach pain or even a life feeling more energetic and healthier all with a simple fix of your diet.

CPSIA information can be obtained
at www.ICGtesting.com
Printed in the USA
BVHW090634270421
605864BV00004B/681